University of CHESTER CAMPUS
Chester LIBRARY
01244 513301

Blackwell
Publishing

Library of Congress Cataloging-in-Publication Data

Fry, Sara T.
Ethics in nursing practice : a guide to ethical decision making / Sara T. Fry, Megan-Jane Johnstone. — 3rd ed.
p. ; cm.
Includes bibliographical references and index.
ISBN-13: 978-1-4051-6052-0 (pbk. : alk. paper)
ISBN-10: 1-4051-6052-7 (pbk. : alk. paper) 1. Nursing ethics. 2. Nursing—Decision making—Moral and ethical aspects. I. Johnstone, Megan-Jane. II. International Council of Nurses. III. Title.
[DNLM: 1. Ethics, Nursing. 2. Decision Making. 3. Ethical Analysis. 4. Nurses—psychology. WY 85 F947e 2008]

RT85.F79 2008
174.2—dc22
2007040792

A catalogue record for this book is available from the British Library.

Set in 10/12.5pt Times NR MT by Graphicraft Limited, Hong Kong
Printed in Singapore by Utopia Press Pte Ltd

1   2008

Contents

Foreword

The first edition of *Ethics in Nursing Practice: A Guide to Ethical Decision Making* was first published in 1994 and a second edition followed in 2002. Over the years this classic textbook has been widely used by nurses and others around the world, and has been translated into several languages including Greek, Italian, Japanese, Korean and Serbian.

I am pleased that the third edition is now available – at a time when ethics and ethical issues have become more complicated, multi-faceted and centre stage in nursing and health. *Ethics in Nursing Practice* is geared to helping nurses and other providers address a wide range of ethical issues. Comprehensive in its coverage of ethics from diverse social, cultural and religious perspectives, and practical in its orientation, *Ethics in Nursing Practice* addresses complex ethical issues and real life dilemmas. It thus guides the reader in ethical decision making and is applicable worldwide.

The International Council of Nurses (ICN) is pleased to again collaborate with Sara T. Fry, RN, PhD, and Megan-Jane Johnstone, RN, PhD, to produce this important resource. The Council and its member national nurses associations have promoted ethics and standards of professional practice as the essence of ICN's mission for more than a century. The Code for Nurses, adopted in 1953 and periodically revised, is at the core of our standards. A cluster of resources – forums, policy statements, guidelines and resolutions – has developed around the Code, and been widely used by nurses everywhere.

This text is a key resource. We are grateful to the authors for this enormous undertaking and contribution to the profession. With the general assistance of staff and the editorial expertise of Blackwell Publishing, they have produced a publication that is scholarly, relevant and practical for a wide audience of practising nurses, managers, teachers, researchers and students.

It is with much pride and high expectations for its use that ICN offers its latest and most comprehensive publication on ethical decision making.

Judith A. Oulton
Chief Executive Officer
International Council of Nurses

Preface

When *The Nurse's Dilemma: Ethical Considerations in Nursing Practice* was published in 1977, the International Council of Nurses took a giant step forward in providing members of the profession worldwide with a guidebook that nurses could use to inform their ethical decision making in complex nursing care situations. The nursing ethics literature was quite meagre at the time; indeed, the field of bioethics was also in its infancy. Nurses, however, were already confronting difficult ethical situations in their practices.

Over the years, nurses' decision making has become increasingly influenced by cultural, religious and political values endemic to the particular situation in which they work. Compounding this influence have been the social, cultural, political and religious factors that have strongly influenced the delivery of healthcare throughout the world and related changes in nursing education and practice. The need for a new guidebook for nurses' ethical decision making to carry the members of the profession into the twenty-first century was satisfied in 1994 by the publication of the first edition of *Ethics in Nursing Practice: A Guide to Ethical Decision Making*. It was the honour and privilege of one of us (S.T.F.), to work with the Professional Services Committee of the ICN in preparing this guidebook for nurses' ethical decision making.

In 2001 revisions to the ICN Code of Ethics for Nurses created a need to update the first edition of *Ethics in Nursing Practice* to reflect the changes made to the Code, changes in ICN position statements and changes in how nurses throughout the world experience ethical issues in practice. To accomplish this task, ICN gathered two nurse ethicists and philosophers – Dr Sara T. Fry, author of the first edition of the guidebook and Professor Megan-Jane Johnstone, a noted nurse ethicist in Australia. Together, this team revised and updated the guidebook in 2002.

Following revision of the ICN Code of Ethics for Nurses in 2006 and additional changes to ICN position statements, Dr Fry and Professor Johnstone agreed to revise and update the guidebook for the third edition. Having completed this task, we are indebted to nurses throughout the world who shared their personal experiences with us and allowed their questions about ethical nursing practice to become part of this book. We received many helpful suggestions for revisions from the ICN staff members, especially Dr Tesfamicael Ghebrehiwet, Consultant, Nursing and Health Policy, and from unknown consultants and readers in several countries. Dr Fry, now retired from nursing education, acknowledges the help of colleagues and friends for their helpful suggestions and support while working on the project. Professor Johnstone acknowledges the Department of Nursing and Midwifery, RMIT University, for its support of the project.

Sara T. Fry *PhD, RN, FAAN*
Formerly Henry R. Luce Professor of Nursing Ethics
Boston College School of Nursing
Chestnut Hill, MA

Megan-Jane Johnstone *BA, PhD, RN, FRCNA*
Professor of Nursing
Division of Nursing and Midwifery
School of Health Sciences
RMIT University, Melbourne

Part 1
Preparation for ethical decision making

Ethical action depends, in part, on the ability of people to recognise that a moral issue exists in a given situation, knowing how to take appropriate ethical action if and when required, and on personal commitment and a genuine desire to achieve moral outcomes (Johnstone 2004). The ability to be able to respond appropriately and effectively to moral issues, in turn, requires development of moral sensitivity, moral reasoning, moral motivation and moral character (Bond 1996; Rest 1986; van Hooft 2006; Wilson 1993). The development and practice of these abilities results in moral behaviour.

Moral sensitivity derives from a person's 'moral sense' (Wilson 1993), and involves awareness of situational aspects that affect the welfare and well-being of an individual. It requires insight, intuition, moral knowing and the ability to recognise the salient moral cues in a given situation to indicate that a moral issue is present. It involves interpreting an individual's verbal and nonverbal behaviours, identifying what he or she wants or needs and responding to him or her in an appropriate manner (Lutzen, Nordstrom & Evertzon 1995; Scott 2006). Moral sensitivity is influenced by one's upbringing, culture, religion, education and life experiences, and may be expressed differently by different people (Lutzen, Johansson & Nordstrom 2000).

Moral reasoning is the act or process of drawing logical conclusions from 'facts' or evidence, and the ability to determine what morally ought to be done in a particular situation. It can involve deciding between conflicting ideals, values or goals in order to decide what one will actually do, or what action one will take to resolve a conflict of values. It is primarily a cognitive process whereby one formulates and justifies an ethically defensible course of action to achieve an ideal moral outcome. Moral reasoning is, however, also informed by intuition and emotion (Damasio 1994; Johnstone 2004).

Moral motivation may be described as a genuine desire and interest to achieve good moral outcomes. It involves deciding between conflicting ideals, values or goals in order to decide what one will actually do, or what action one will take to resolve a conflict of values. It involves one's sense of moral responsibility and integrity, and a commitment to achieving moral ends (Peter, Lunardi & Macfarlane 2004). It often includes a view of oneself as a fair, honourable, morally competent and self-respecting person.

Moral character is the perseverance, strength of conviction and courage that enables a person to carry out a plan of moral action that he or she has deemed morally imperative. Together, these abilities represent what it takes for one to act morally (van Hooft 2006).

Learning about codes of ethics, standards for ethical practice in nursing, concepts of ethics and value formation, helps the nurse to develop his or her abilities to be moral and to integrate them with problem-solving skills gained in earlier education and in nursing practice. As these abilities are repeatedly used to confront complex ethical issues in patient care, they are refined and sharpened over time. Their development leads to ethical behaviours and ethical decision-making excellence.

Part 1 defines and describes the nature of value formation and value conflicts (Chapter 1), the discipline of ethics (Chapter 2), basic ethical concepts of nursing practice (Chapter 3), standards for ethical behaviours such as principles, rules and codes of ethics (Chapter 4) and the application of ethical analysis and ethical action to patient care situations (Chapter 5). Case examples demonstrate the moral behaviours and ethical decisions of nurses in different social, cultural and political environments when confronted with complex ethical issues in patient care.

Chapter 1
Value formation and value conflict

Case example 1: The director of nursing who valued organisation

Mr Williams has worked in a nursing home for three years. Recently, a new director of nursing was appointed, a very efficient person who wants everybody and everything to be organised. For example, she insists that all patients be bathed before breakfast even though some patients would rather wait until after breakfast. The patients tell Mr Williams that they are very unhappy with this new rule. Mr Williams understands the patients' point of view but fears that the new director of nursing will think he is insubordinate if he questions the new rule requiring all patients be bathed before breakfast. He needs his job to support his family.

Case example 2: Valuing maternal/child care above anything else

Mrs Kenoba is the nurse supervisor of a hospital in a small industrial city. There are many childbearing families served by the hospital. While nursing services are adequate for normal birthing and the care of full term babies, there are limited services for obstetrical emergencies and premature infants. Mrs Kenoba would like to divert the majority of her nursing resources to provide more nursing attention to the mothers who are sickest and to the low birth weight infants. The hospital administration, however, objects to her plans. Given the depressed economic situation in the city, the hospital executive believes that it should provide care to those who are healthiest, most likely to return to work quickly and who can most contribute to the economy of the community. Mrs Kenoba, however, is uncomfortable with this decision.

Case example 3: Being asked to assist in an abortion

Mrs Camino has been asked to assist in an abortion. The patient is a young un-married woman who has come to the hospital without family members or friends. Mrs Camino does not want to assist in the procedure because her religious beliefs view abortion as the killing of a human being and not permissible. She tells the physician that she will find another nurse to assist him. The physician, however, wants to begin the procedure immediately, and becomes very angry when Mrs Camino refuses to help him. He threatens to report her to the nurse supervisor.

Every nurse makes countless decisions about patient care including what care to give, when to give it, where it should be given, how it should be given and by whom. Each decision requires the nurse to consider information about the patient in the context of values – personal, patient, individual, communal, cultural and professional – to determine how best to care for the patient or assist the patient in self-care. Factual information about the patient comes from many sources: the healthcare record, the results of diagnostic tests, the nursing assessment and the patient's history as supplied by the patient, the patient's family, or other primary carers including close friends. Information alone, however, cannot help the nurse decide what he or she should do to provide 'ethical' care for the patient. To decide what is ethically right to do in nursing care, one must consider information about the patient within a framework or context of values (Fry & Veatch 2006).

The nature of values

Values, in a sociological sense, may be defined as those 'things of social life' (ideals, customs and institutions) toward which people have an 'affective regard' (*Macquarie Dictionary* 2006). Values in this sense may be either positive or negative. For example, a person or group of people may hold positive values about freedom, birthday celebrations and education, but negative values about cruelty, crime and conscription. In contrast, values in a moral sense pertain to the quality of things (decisions, actions, behaviours) that are desirable for moral reasons. A theory of values, in turn, is 'a theory about what things in the world are good, desirable and important' (Flew & Priest 2002, p. 415).

Values often arise from needs or wants (Glen 1999) and are derived from many sources such as a person's culture, family, peer group or work environment. They can be easily identified in the everyday life experiences of a person and can be inferred indirectly from that person's verbal and nonverbal behaviours. They can be expressed in language or in standards of conduct that a person endorses or tries to maintain. Values are organised into a system that has meaning to the individual. This system of values represents the individual's set of beliefs about what he or she believes to be true (Rokeach 1973). Some values are more import-ant than others and are prioritised higher within an individual's value system.

This hierarchy is usually fairly stable over time but other values can and do replace higher values based on life experiences and an individual's reassessment of his values (Rokeach 1973).

Once part of the person's value system, any value can have motivational power and guide that person's choices. Unfortunately, individuals are often unaware of the values that motivate their choices and decisions. As a result, understanding one's values is the first step in preparing oneself to make ethical decisions.

It is important to note that values may be of a nonmoral or moral nature. The two are differentiated below.

Nonmoral values

Some of the values held by the nurse are nonmoral, that is, they are not of a moral nature. They are values that are not based on moral considerations and the significant moral interests of people. Like style and decorum, they are values related to personal preferences, beliefs or matters of taste (Frankena 1973). In Case example 1, the new nursing supervisor values organisation and the practice of early bathing of patients, considering these more important than patient choice of times for bathing. For her, the rules about early bathing of patients, organisation and efficiency are nonmorally good because they represent matters of taste, efficiency, routine and order.

Moral values

Moral values are of a distinctively moral nature in that they derive from the significant moral interests people have in upholding such things as human life, freedom and self-determination, welfare and well-being. Ethics is largely about the processes we use to ascribe moral values to human actions, behaviours, institutions or character traits (Frankena 1973) and, in turn, justify those ascriptions. In Case example 3, Mrs Camino values the protection of human fetal life. Not aborting human fetal life is morally good for Mrs Camino because it is an action that, in her view, preserves human life and has moral implications for how humans regard human life through all its stages.

Cultural values

Cultural values are the accepted and dominant standards of a particular cultural group. They function in conjunction with belief systems and serve to give meaning and worth to the existence and experiences of the group. Cultural values and standards (together with beliefs) play a significant role in shaping a group's customs and traditions (including religious practices). They may also define the acceptable and nonacceptable behaviours of group members, as well as prescribe social relationships and rules of communication among group members. The group's moral order and indeed, 'the whole spirit and web of meaning and purpose of a given group in a particular place and time' may stem from cultural values (Kanitsaki 1994, p. 95).

All cultures have a moral system and moral values and beliefs about what constitutes 'right' and 'wrong' conduct. Similarly, all cultures have principles and rules which can be appealed to for guiding morally just conduct. However, just what these principles and rules are, how they are defined, applied, and who ultimately applies them varies across, and even within, different cultures (Johnstone 2004).

Every culture has values and beliefs about health and illness and about what is morally acceptable behaviour in the provision of health-promoting care to people. As with moral rules of conduct, however, how health and illness are defined and interpreted, what constitutes acceptable and therapeutically effective care, when care should be provided, where (location and context), and by whom, varies across, and within, different cultures (Jormsri, Kunaviktikul, Ketefian & Chaowalit 2005; Kanitsaki 1994; Lutzen 1997).

Some cultures, such as the Anglo-American cultures, place a high value on the sovereignty of the individual and the rights of individuals to make choices about their lives free from the interference of others (including family and friends). Other cultures, for example the cultures of indigenous peoples of colonised countries, traditional Greek and Italian cultures and many of the traditional cultural groups found in South Asia, place a high value on the family, collective and communal decision making and the overriding obligation of individual family members to place the interests of their family above their own (Johnstone 2004; Long 1999). Culture, however, is not static and many people may adopt and exhibit values that are characteristic of different and sometimes competing cultural life ways. This is especially so in the case of people who are bi-cultural, those who share meaningful membership of two cultural groups, or those who are 'multi-cultural', those who share membership of more than one cultural group, including sub-cultural groups.

It is important to understand that every culture has a system of ethics. It is also important to understand that every ethical system is the product of the culture and history from which it has emerged. Nevertheless, it is possible and imperative for nurses to understand the nature of cultural differences (and similarities) and how different cultural values can influence attitudes, beliefs, caring practices, decision making and the behaviours of people (lay and professional) in healthcare contexts (Doswell & Erlen 1998; Grabbe 2000; Imes & Landry 2002). For example, in some traditional cultures, death of the elderly is seen to be unjust; in some more contemporary cultures, death of the elderly is seen to be expected and even a 'blessing' at the end of a life well lived. Some cultures may place a high value on the health-promoting behaviours of physical exercise; other cultures may, however, regard more passive behaviours such as meditation more conducive to promoting health. Just as it is important to understand that every culture has a system of ethics, so too is it important to understand that every ethical system is the product of its own culture and history. Since nursing is practised in many different cultural systems, any discussion of ethics must consider the values underpinning and expressed by the culture of the population cared for, and how those values relate to proposed nursing interventions (Bodell & Weng 2000; Chen 2001; Moazam 2000; Tangwa 2000). Nurses also need to be mindful that the moral rules and principles of one culture cannot always be applied appropriately, reliably or meaningfully to another culture – at least, not without modification (Johnstone 2004).

Religious values

Religious values (often confused with cultural values and beliefs and/or the culture of a people) are, like ethics, the product of the culture and history from which they have emerged. Not all people grow up under the influence of an organised religion. Many do however, and many continue to practise a religious faith throughout their lives.

The values learned in a religious context are very powerful and enduring, and can continue to influence people's attitudes and beliefs even when they have 'abandoned' a particular religious belief system.

Religious values can be acted out unconsciously by individuals. This is because religious values are often deeply embedded in the background and experience of the person (that is, 'embodied') and cannot be called into question without questioning that person's own concept of 'self'. For example, most religions adhere to certain tenets that influence individuals' beliefs concerning life and death and the importance of the afterlife. In Case example 3, Mrs Camino expresses the importance of her religious values by deciding not to assist the physician in an abortion. If she had assisted in the abortion, the act would have violated her beliefs and undermined her concept of herself as a moral person.

The teachings of many organised religions seek to embrace almost every aspect of human activity. For example, in each aspect of Orthodox Judaism there are specific values and principles which are usually embodied in specific laws including those governing food preparation (Berkovits 1990). Hinduism is a diverse set of religious and philosophical beliefs that gives spiritual meaning to individual attitudes and actions toward others (Thompson 2003). Islam requires its adherents (Muslims) to submit themselves to the will of Allah in all aspects of living. The geographic mobility of modern society means that nurses may care for patients with cultural values and religious beliefs very different from their own; values and beliefs that must be acknowledged and respected in order to provide effective care (Imes & Landry 2002; Papadopoulos 2006; Yeh 2001).

Personal values

Personal values are informed by individual beliefs, attitudes, standards and ideals that guide behaviour and how a person experiences life. For example, one person may value excellence and strive to achieve excellence in all that he or she does while another person may be content to be average. One nurse may person-ally value cleanliness (a nonmoral value) and value honesty (a moral value). Personal values will be important to the nurse and will influence the kinds of judg-ments he or she makes. They may also influence the kinds of behaviours/actions the nurse takes. A person's values are arranged in a hierarchy based on import-ance to that individual. Personal value systems can vary widely from person to person, thus it can never be assumed that another's personal value system is similar to yours (Gallagher & Boyd 1991; Wronska & Marianiski 2002).

Each nurse has a personal value system influenced by his or her upbringing, culture, religious and political beliefs, education and life experiences. As Barrett (1990, pp. 17–19) points out:

> 'The society in which we live and the societal influences within it promote and uphold certain values. Development of values can be facilitated through exchange of attitudes and beliefs. In nursing, this can occur through role model-ling and the education process . . . Values and value systems are a guiding force, consciously or subconsciously.'

Identifying the values in one's own value system through introspection and self-reflection is an essential aspect of ethical decision making.

Another aspect of ethical decision making is understanding values that are important to other individuals and the reasons why they are important (Fry & Veatch 2006). Each person prioritises his or her values differently, based on his or her belief system and hierarchy of values. Understanding the value systems of others, and acknowledging and respecting that they are equally as valid as one's own value system, is essential to making ethical decisions.

Professional values

Professional values relate to the ultimate standards that have been agreed to, and are expected to be upheld by a professional group (Johnstone 1998). Pro-fessional values in nursing are those promoted by the professional codes of ethics, professional codes of conduct, professional competence standards (see, for example, ANMC 2008) and the practice of nursing. Nurses learn about pro-fessional values both from formal instruction and from informal observation of practising nurses, and gradually incorporate professional values into their personal value system.

Some traditional professional values of nursing are nonmoral, that is, based on personal preference or taste and social prescriptions of style and decorum. Examples include: dress codes (including the colour and style of uniforms), clean-liness, established routine ('we have always done it this way') and efficiency, to name a few (Johnstone 2004). Other professional values are distinctly moral in nature, for example: integrity, justice, fairness, care, compassion, honesty, verac-ity, fidelity, advocacy, compassion and the like. In Case example 2, Mrs Kenoba expresses professional values when she desires to distribute nursing resources to those patients who are the sickest and in greatest need of nursing services. The fact that she is not permitted to do so indicates that other values are considered more important, in this situation, than these professional values.

Professional values are made explicit in a code of ethics, a code of conduct and other formal statements that establish and make public the standards of a professional group. For example, the International Council of Nurses (ICN) *Code of Ethics for Nurses* (2006a, p. 1) reflects professional values in its statement, 'Inherent in nursing is respect for human rights, including the right to life, to dignity and to be treated with respect'. The preface to the American Nurses Association *Code of Ethics for Nurses* states that 'A code of ethics makes explicit the primary goals, values, and obligations of the profession' (2001, p. 5). Each point of the Canadian Nurses' Association *Code of Ethics for Registered Nurses* (2002) is stated as a value and is followed by descriptions of the required nursing obligations to honour the value. The Australian Nursing & Midwifery Council's *Code of Ethics for Nurses in Australia* (2008) states 'This Code contains eight value statements, and nurses and students of nursing are encouraged to use these as a guide when reflecting upon the degree to which their clinical, managerial, educational, or research practice demonstrates & upholds these values'. The New Zealand Nurses Organisation (NZNO) *Code of Ethics* (2001) lists professional values relating to clients, the healthcare team, the social context of nursing practice and the professional association. Codes of nursing ethics make public the professional values of nursing and indicate the values central to professional education programmes.

Value conflicts

Both moral and nonmoral values can easily conflict with one another and with patients' rights and nurses' professional duties. Personal values may conflict with professional values, which in turn may conflict with cultural values. The nurse's value of doing good to the patient might conflict with her value of honouring the patient's choices or his or her right to make such choices. The nurse's value of giving safe medication dosages might conflict with the patient's value of relief from pain and the perceived professional duty to relieve suffering. The elderly resident's value of personal liberty and being able to walk freely around an aged care facility at any time, both day and night, might conflict with the institution's value of client safety, achieved by surveillance and security locks on all public thoroughfares leading to and from the facility.

In each of these situations, the nurse must first identify the values involved, the strength and relevance of rights claimed and their corresponding duties, and where a conflict between values, rights and/or duties may be occurring. The nurse must then make a decision based on which values are most important and which rights claims are most warranted and deserving of respect. When moral values, rights claims and associated duties are involved, resolving value conflict becomes a complex and sometimes perplexing ethical decision-making process.

In Case example 1, Mr Williams values respecting patients' choices concerning their care and the increased well-being of his patients. He understands that the patients' preferences concerning bathing times conflict with those of the nursing supervisor (a nonmoral conflict) and that following the new rule will diminish their sense of well-being (a moral conflict). Although he feels obliged as a professional to increase the patients' sense of well-being (a personal and professional value), he is also influenced by his need to provide for his family (a personal and cultural value). He must decide which of these values are most important to him and what the practice of nursing requires in terms of promoting the significant moral interests of the patients and honouring professional values. Before he can decide, however, he must clarify the values and significant moral interests of all parties involved and honestly explore the importance of these values and interests to him. This is the first step of making an ethical decision and its importance cannot be overestimated.

In Case example 2, Mrs Kenoba is experiencing a value conflict with her hospital administration's directions concerning assignment of nursing staff. Mrs Kenoba values providing care to those who are sickest and have the greatest need of nursing services (a personal and professional value). The hospital administration values providing services to those who can most profit from the time, money and resources invested in their care (a social and political value). Since Mrs Kenoba is a member of the social and political community as well as a nurse, she must examine the importance of her personal and professional values and decide how to honour them while also honouring the values of her employer.

In Case example 3, Mrs Camino faces a conflict between the professional value of providing nursing care to those in need of services and her personal values concerning abortion which are based on her religious beliefs. Although Mrs Camino seems to be aware of her values based on religious beliefs, she needs to examine whether these values can override the giving of basic nursing care when that care would go against her conscience. It may not seem right that any patient should go without nursing care simply because the religious belief system of the nurse does not permit the nurse to give that type of nursing care. Yet, no nurse should be expected to provide nursing care against his or her conscience (Johnstone 2004). How can this conflict of values be resolved?

Fortunately, professional nursing guidelines and codes of ethics provide direction for this type of value conflict. Nurses usually are obliged to provide care to a patient whose personal values and belief systems may differ from their own, especially when no other nurse is available to care for the patient. The nurse's primary responsibility is to people requiring nursing care (ICN 2006a) and those in need of care have a right to receive care and not be discriminated against on the basis of race, ethnicity, religious beliefs or other personal characteristics (ICN 2006b; WHO 2002). This right includes the right to choose, or decline, nursing care (Dudzinski & Shannon 2006). It also includes the right to accept or refuse medical treatment, to waive informed consent and confidentiality, and the right to dignity and to die with dignity. Where nurses face a 'dual loyalty' involving conflicts between their professional duties and their obligations to their employer or other authority, the nurse's primary responsibility is to those who require care (ICN 2006a, p. 1).

Summary

The first task, in preparing for ethical decision making, is to consider the values both of the nurse and of the patient. Every nurse is influenced by his or her own value system, shaped over time by culture, religion, education and life experiences. Patients also have value systems that may differ significantly from the value system of the nurse. Understanding the nature of moral and nonmoral values helps the nurse determine the relative importance of cultural, religious, personal, professional and other values in everyday nursing practice. When values conflict with one another, the nurse needs to respect the values of others, balancing value considerations in relation to patients' rights and the nurses' professional duties.

References

American Nurses Association (2001) *Code of ethics for nurses with interpretive statements*. Washington, DC: ANA.

Australian Nursing & Midwifery Council (ANMC) (2008) *Code of ethics for nurses in Australia*. Canberra: ANMC.

Barrett, E.M. (1990) A philosophy of nursing. *I.N.F. & H.S.* November/December, 17–19.

Berkovits, B. (1990) A Jewish perspective on nursing. *Nurs Stand* 4(28), 32–34.

Bodell, J. & Weng, M.A. (2000) The Jewish patient and terminal dehydration: A hospice ethical dilemma. *Amer J Hospice & Palliative Care* 17(3), 185–188.

Bond, E.J. (1996) *Ethics and human well-being*. Cambridge, Mass: Blackwell Publishers.

Canadian Nurses' Association (2002) *Code of ethics for registered nurses*. Ottawa, Ontario: CNA.

Chen, Y.C. (2001) Chinese values, health and nursing. *J Adv Nurs* 36(2), 270–273.

Damasio, A. (1994) *Descartes error: Emotion, reason, and the human brain*. New York: Avon Books.

Doswell, W.M. & Erlen, J.A. (1998) Multicultural issues and ethical concerns in the delivery of nursing care interventions. *Nurs Clin N Amer* 33(2), 353–361.

Dudzinski, D. & Shannon, S. (2006) Competent patients' refusal of nursing care. *Nurs Ethics* 13(6), 608–621.

Flew, A. & Priest, S. (Eds) (2002) *A dictionary of philosophy*. London: Pan Books.

Frankena, W. (1973) *Ethics*, 2nd ed. Englewood Cliffs, NJ: Prentice Hall.

Fry, S.T. & Veatch R.M. (2006) *Case studies in nursing ethics*, 3rd ed. Boston: Jones & Bartlett.

Gallagher, U. & Boyd, K.M. (1991) *Teaching and learning nursing ethics*. Middlesex, England: Scutari Press.

Glen, S. (1999) Educating for interprofessional collaboration: Teaching about values. *Nurs Ethics* 6(3), 202–213.

Grabbe, L. (2000) Understanding patients from the former Soviet Union. *Inter Fam Medicine* 32(3), 201–206.

Imes, S. & Landry, D. (2002) Don't underestimate the power of culture. *SCI Nurs* 19(4), 172–176.

International Council of Nurses (ICN) (2006a) *Code of ethics for nurses*. Geneva, Switzerland: ICN.

International Council of Nurses (ICN) (2006b) *ICN position statement: Nurses and human rights*. Geneva, Switzerland: ICN.

Johnstone, M.-J. (1998) *Determining and responding effectively to ethical professional misconduct in nursing: A report to the Nurses Board of Victoria*. Melbourne: RMIT University.

Johnstone, M.-J. (2004) *Bioethics: A nursing perspective*, 4th ed. Sydney: Elsevier Science.

Jormsri, P., Kunaviktikul W., Ketefian, S. & Chaowalit, A. (2005) Moral competence to nursing practice. *Nurs Ethics* 12(6), 582–594.

Kanitsaki, O. (1994) Cultural and linguistic diversity. In J. Romanini and J. Daly (Eds) *Critical care nursing: Australian perspectives*. Sydney: Baillière Tindall/W.B. Saunders.

Long, S.O. (1999) Family surrogacy and cancer disclosure: Physician–family negotiation of an ethical dilemma in Japan. *J Palliative Care* 15(3), 31–42.

Lutzen, K. (1997) Nursing ethics into the next millennium: A context-sensitive approach for nursing ethics. *Nurs Ethics* 4(3), 218–226.

Lutzen, K., Nordstrom, G. & Evertzon, M. (1995) Moral sensitivity in nursing practice. *Scand J Caring Sci* 9(3), 131–138.

Lutzen, K., Johansson, A. & Nordstrom, G. (2000) Moral sensitivity: Some differences between nurses and physicians. *Nurs Ethics* 7(6), 520–530.

Macquarie Dictionary, 4th ed. (2006) Macquarie, NSW: Macquarie University.

Moazam, F. (2000) Families, patients, and physicians in medical decisionmaking: A Pakistani perspective. *Hastings Center Rep* 30(6), 28–37.

New Zealand Nurses Organisation (2001) *Code of ethics*. Wellington, New Zealand: NZNO.

Papadopolous, I. (2006) *Transcultural health and social care: Development of culturally competent practitioners*. Edinburgh: Elsevier/Churchill Livingstone.

Peter, E., Lunardi, V.L. & Macfarlane, A. (2004) Nursing resistance as ethical action: Literature review. *J Adv Nurs* 46(4), 403–416.

Rest, J. (1986) *Moral development: Advances in research and theory*. New York: Wiley.

Rokeach, M. (1973) *The nature of human values*. New York: Free Press.

Scott, P.A. (2006) Perceiving the moral dimension of practice: Insights from Murdoch, Vetiesen, and Aristotle. *Nurs Philos* 7(3), 137–145.

Tangwa, G.B. (2000) The traditional African perception of a person. *Hastings Center Rep* 30(5), 39–43.

Thompson, M. (2003) *Eastern philosophy*. London: Hodder Arnold.

van Hooft S. (2006) *Understanding virtue ethics*. Chesham, Bucks UK: Acumen Publishing Ltd.

Varcoe, C., Doane, G., Pauly, B., Rodney, P., Storch, J.L., Mahoney, K., McPherson, G., Brown, H. & Starzomski, R. (2004) Ethical practice in nursing: Working the in-betweens. *J Adv Nurs* 45(3), 316–325.

Wilson, J.Q. (1993) *The moral sense*. New York: Free Press.

World Health Organization (WHO) (2002) *25 questions and answers on health and human rights*. Health and human rights publication series, issue no. 1, Geneva: WHO.

Wronska, I. & Marianiski, J. (2002) The fundamental values of nurses in Poland. *Nurs Ethics* 9(1), 92–100.

Yeh, C.H. (2001) Religious beliefs and practices of Taiwanese parents of pediatric patients with cancer. *Cancer Nurs* 24(6), 476–482.

Chapter 2
The discipline of ethics

It is important to comprehend the frameworks and traditions that guide ethics inquiry, in general, and nursing ethics, in particular. This chapter provides an overview of the frameworks and traditions that have guided ethics inquiry, the development of bioethics (i.e. ethics inquiry in the biomedical sciences), and nursing ethics.

The word ethics has several meanings, all of which relate to the standards that govern conduct or behaviour. Ethics is sometimes confused with etiquette, that is, standards of style and decorum valued by a particular group. In the past, what was often taught to nurses as professional ethics was really professional etiquette, and had more to do with teaching nurses to be obedient servants than reflective moral practitioners (Johnstone 2004).

In the field of moral philosophy, ethics is generally understood to be a system of action-guiding principles and rules which function by specifying the types of conduct that are permitted (allowed), required (obligatory) and forbidden (never allowed) (Johnstone 2004). Ethics also involves a systematic examination of the moral life and seeks to provide sound justification for the moral decisions and actions of people (Beauchamp & Childress 2001). Ethical systems and related processes can be either secular or religious (theological) in origin and nature. Ethics can be examined and applied from a particular or general perspective, and in a personal or public way. For example, the expression of an ethical point of view can be of a personal and highly individual nature (e.g. personal ethics) or be of a more public and collective nature (e.g. professional ethics – such as professional medical ethics, professional nursing ethics, etc). In either case, standards of conduct are at issue.

Personal ethics can be appropriately described as the personal set of moral values which an individual chooses to live by and which generally guide his or her approach to their moral life and relationships with others. Matters of conscience are a good example of personal morality (Johnstone 2004), although these may also accord with professional ethics. Professional ethics can be described as the agreed standards and behaviours expected of members of a given professional group and that are prescribed in that group's code of professional conduct. For example, nurses are expected to maintain certain standards of ethical conduct in professional activities. These standards are usually prescribed in their professional codes of ethics (such as the International Council of Nurses' *Code of Ethics for Nurses* 2006) and may be supported by law.

The word ethics can also refer to the type of philosophical inquiry that helps us understand the moral dimensions of human conduct. In this sense, ethics examines what is right or wrong to do, or what is good or bad human conduct.

Throughout this book, the term ethics is used in all of the ways described above. That is, ethics is used to refer to the moral practices and beliefs of health professionals, the particular moral standards of a single group of professionals (nurses, physicians, etc.), as well as the type of inquiry about the principles of ethics (both secular and religious). Ethical inquiry helps us to understand the moral dimensions of human conduct and to formulate our responses to significant questions about human well-being (Fry & Veatch 2006; Johnstone 2004).

For the purposes of this book, the term nursing ethics refers to philosophical inquiry about the moral dimensions of nursing practice. It involves analysis of the moral phenomena found in nursing practice and the moral language and moral foundations of nursing practice (Fry 2004a). It includes analysis of ethical judgments made by nurses (Fry & Veatch 2006). Nursing ethics also includes the examination of ethical and bioethical issues from the perspectives of nursing theory and practice (Johnstone 2004).

Traditional western ethics

Traditional western ethics is characterised by subject matter, methods, theories and principles, as described below. Twenty-first century ethics discourse and ethics literature have been strongly influenced by traditional western ethics and its approaches.

Subject matter of ethics

Ethics can focus on one of several forms or areas of inquiry, three of which are mentioned below. Normative ethics examines the standards (norms) or criteria

Utilitarianism – Theory that maintains that the moral rightness of actions is determined by the balance of good and bad consequences of those actions. Desired consequences are an increase in positive value produced by the action (increase in pleasure, health, friendship or knowledge, for example). (Example: Jeremy Bentham or John Stuart Mill)

Naturalism – Theory that maintains that humankind has been created with identifiable tendencies toward certain values. These tendencies include the inclination toward community, respect for the rights of others, honesty and a just government. Ethical principles and rules about what people ought to do are derived from these tendencies. (Example: Saint Thomas Aquinas or John Calvin)

Formalism – Theory that maintains that the moral rightness of actions is determined by their nature or their form. Desired nature and form includes the keeping of duties or special obligations (parent to child) and following certain rules (keeping a promise, for example). Actions are morally significant if their form honours duty or follows the principle/rule. (Example: Immanuel Kant)

Pragmatism – Theory that maintains that moral rightness of actions is determined by what works or is most useful. Desired results are those that are practically significant or that serve a useful function. An action has moral meaning or value if it is practically significant (Example: William James)

Figure 2.1   Common moral theories used in normative ethics.

for right or wrong conduct (Frankena 1973). Using ethical theories such as utilitarianism, naturalism, formalism and pragmatism (Figure 2.1), it defends a system of moral principles and rules to determine which actions are right or wrong. In this form of inquiry, the moral importance of perceived duties and obligations in human interaction are assessed and theories of moral human conduct are used to support one normative position rather than another.

Nonnormative ethics includes two forms of inquiry: descriptive ethics and metaethics. Descriptive ethics investigates and explains the phenomena of moral beliefs and behaviour (Frankena 1973). Those who investigate the moral reasoning patterns and moral judgments of nurses are usually engaged in descriptive ethics (Ketefian & Fry 1998).

Metaethics concerns the analysis of moral language and concepts used in ethics inquiry and the logic of moral justification (Beauchamp & Childress 2001; Jecker, Jonsen & Pearlman 2007). It is a secondary level of inquiry that provides theories about ethics rather than theories for ethical conduct. Typical metaethical investigations consider the connections between human conduct and morality, the connections between ethical beliefs (values) and the facts of the real world, and the relationships among ethical theories, principles, rules and human conduct. Inquiry about the moral language of nursing (advocacy, accountability, cooperation and caring) falls within the area of metaethics as well.

These forms of ethical inquiry are closely related and their interactions yield a system of applied ethics (Figure 2.2). For example, one might first use descriptive ethics to describe a moral phenomenon (such as the protection of patients from harm), then use normative ethics to argue for the moral accountability of the nurse in patient care, and finally use metaethics to explain the meaning of

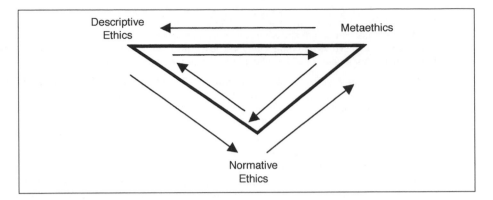

Figure 2.2   Applied ethics.

accountability within nursing practice. The results of this process could then be applied to a particular patient care situation (see also Johnstone 1998).

Methods of ethics

Various methods can be used to investigate and evaluate morality, our culturally defined moral goals and the rules governing how we attain these goals (see, for example, Jecker, Jonsen & Pearlman 2007). Since ethics is a form of philosophical inquiry, one of the most common methods is argumentation. Four types of argumentation are described below.

One type of argument often used by ethicists is called 'the appeal to authority' (Ladd 1978), which states that one ought, or ought not, to do some action because authority tells us to do so. The authority appealed to may be another person (e.g. mother, father, priest), a group of persons (e.g. the profession of nursing), an institution (e.g. a church or a health agency) or even a hypothetical person (e.g. the patient, members of society). The effectiveness of this method of argumentation depends on individual belief and faith in the authority cited.

A second type of argument is called 'the appeal to consensus' (Ladd 1978), which cites the supposed agreement of people (or groups of people) on an issue to establish its particular ethical position. Like the first method, it relies on individual belief and faith in the people (or groups of people) who agree on the issue.

A third method of argument is the 'appeal to intuition' (Ladd 1978), a method with a long tradition in ethics dating back to the Pythagorean cults of Ancient Greece. This form of argument asserts that at least some moral judgments are known to be true by intuition, and that moral intuition is a valid form of ethical knowledge. It is meaningful, however, only with persons who also rely on ethical intuition. Not everyone subscribes to this view. Some reject its assertions on the grounds that since intuitions change over time, they cannot be trusted to be a reliable guide to moral action. In addition, the circumstances or conditions that gave rise to the intuition may change. These objections, however, equally apply to ethical rationalism (that ethics is known to be true by way of reason) and the other forms of ethical argument discussed here. Nevertheless, it is always important to know whether an ethical argument is being advanced solely on the basis of intuition rather than other forms of argument. Today, intuition is being increasingly recognised as an important ingredient of sound clinical and moral decision making (Damasio 1994; Davis-Floyd & Arvidson 1997; King & Clark 2002).

The fourth and last type of argument is called the 'dialectic' or 'Socratic' method (Ladd 1978). It begins by asking questions and then considering answers that are supported by good reasons and logical thought. It enjoys a long and respected tradition in ethics and relies on reason or rationality for its strength.

It is important to note the types of arguments used in making ethical judgments. Any ethical judgment must be supported by sound argument. However, results of arguments may differ depending on the type of argument advanced. Since ethical judgments often serve as a basis for individual actions, one must make sure that the method of argumentation used to reach a judgment is ethically valid and has been correctly followed. This is particularly important in normative ethics but may influence metaethical investigations, as well.

Ethics and justification

Before moving on to discuss the theories of ethics, it would be useful at this point to provide some explanation of the role of ethics and ethical theory in justifying – that is, providing the strongest moral reasons for – our moral decisions and actions.

Ethics, as we have seen, is concerned with value judgments and, in particular, with value judgments about 'right' and 'wrong', 'good' and 'bad' behaviour. It is important to understand, however, that ethics is not just about identifying or ascribing (giving) the values of good or bad/right or wrong to certain people, decisions and actions. Another critical role of ethics is to provide sound justification for the value judgments we make.

Moral conflict and disagreements occur often in healthcare contexts. Given the complexity of the values that operate in healthcare domains it is not surprising that people may express moral values, beliefs and evaluations which are not shared by others or which others do not agree with (Johnstone 2004).

When experiencing situations involving moral disagreement and conflict it is tempting for decision makers to rely on their own personal values and beliefs about what constitutes right and wrong behaviour. But personal preferences or our own 'ordinary moral apparatus' may not be reliable guides to moral conduct. As Kopelman (1995, p. 117) warns, our own personal views can result from 'prejudice, self-interest or ignorance' and thus may lead us to make 'moral mistakes'. Because of this we need to look elsewhere to strengthen the warranties – that is, to justify or find very strong reasons to support – our moral choices and actions. Ethical theory is generally regarded as the ultimate source from where such warranties or very strong reasons (justifications) can be found (Johnstone 2004).

When dealing with moral disagreement or addressing ethical issues in practice, it is essential that nurses *justify* their moral decisions and actions, that is, that they provide the strongest moral reasons behind them (Beauchamp & Childress 2001). However, a number of questions arise here:

> 'How do we decide if the reasons we offer for [our] appraisals are good reasons? What is the *ground* for our decision that some reasons are good reasons and others are not? When, if at all, can we say that these grounds are sufficient for our moral decisions?' (Nielsen 1989, p. 53, emphasis original).

Beauchamp & Childress (2001, p. 385) suggest three possible answers to these questions:

(1) moral rules, principles and theories
(2) lived experience and individuated personal judgments
(3) a combination (synthesis) of both these (theoretical and experiential) approaches

Beauchamp & Childress's reference to lived experience and individuated personal judgment should not be interpreted to mean that personal judgments can and should override ethical considerations. Ultimately, ethical rules, principles and theories provide the foundations of and justifications needed for ethical decision making and conduct. Nevertheless, lived experience and individuated personal judgments are also crucial to the appropriate selection, interpretation, cultural adaptation and application of relevant ethical rules, principles and theories. In practice, theory and practice function as a two-way process with each informing the other. Applied to nursing, this means ethical rules, principles and theories inform nursing practice, and at the same time, nursing practice informs ethical rules, principles and theories.

Theories of ethics

There are many ways to classify theories of ethics. Some theories are classical, implying a rich historical tradition and concern with the 'good life' or how to achieve the 'good life'. Examples of classical theories of ethics are hedonism (pleasure is the sole good of human life), and stoicism (indifference to pleasure or pain). Other theories of ethics are considered modern in that they apply philosophical analysis to ethical conduct in order to find out the meaning of terms and statements that appear in theories. Examples of modern analytical theories of ethics are naturalism (moral judgments are true or false and can be reduced to a concept of natural science), emotivism (moral judgments cannot be verified or falsified by scientific procedures; they are simply judgments about one's feelings) and intuitionism (people know the meaning of our moral terms and principles because we see them in human experience and can grasp their significance as an intuitive act).

Another way to classify theories of ethics is to consider them 'western' or 'eastern'. Western theories of ethics are based on European or American philosophies, and are often influenced by Judaeo-Christian systems of beliefs (Jecker, Jonsen & Pearlman 2007). Examples of western theories of ethics are utilitarianism, naturalism, formalism and pragmatism (Figure 2.1). Eastern theories of ethics are based on Asian, Indian or Arabic philosophies, and may also be influenced by religious systems of belief (Thompson 2003). One example of an eastern theory of ethics is Confucianism. In its earliest form, Confucianism was a system of ethical precepts for the proper management of society (Nyitay 2004). It viewed the human being as essentially a social creature, bound to others by *jen*, a term often interpreted as sympathy or human benevolence. Jen is expressed through the five relations – sovereign and subject, parent and child, elder and younger sibling, husband and wife, and friend and friend. Of these relations, filial piety or *hsiao* is emphasised. The relations function smoothly by adhering to a combination of etiquette and ritual. Correct conduct proceeds not through compulsion, but through a sense of virtue developed by observing suitable models of ethical behaviour.

Other theories of ethics are derived from Buddhism, Hinduism and Islam. Buddhist ethics directs devotees of Buddha to refrain from killing, stealing, lying, sexual misconduct and use of intoxicants (Saddhatissa 1987). Devotees are also urged to cultivate the virtues of friendliness (to disarm hostility), compassion (to remove the suffering of others), sympathetic joy (to rejoice in the success of others), and equanimity (to be even-handed with regard to the actions of others) (Harvey 2000). Buddhists' responses to contemporary ethical issues in healthcare are based on the Buddhist view of the universe, the nature of humanity and belief in impermanence. Hindu ethics emphasises principles of righteous conduct and the doctrine of transmigration where, at physical death, the soul (or self) is carried to another body in which it flourishes or suffers according to previous behaviour (Coward, Lipner & Young 1989). The three aims of life for the Hindu are to achieve dharma (adherence to religious and ethical norms in order to ensure a happier rebirth), artha (building up wealth for the benefit of oneself and one's family) and kama (seeking pleasure and the satisfaction of personal desires) (Weiss 2004). Virtues such as honesty, hospitality and generosity are also encouraged. Islamic ethics are likewise based on religious teachings. The five essential religious and moral duties of Muslims are to:

(1) profess faith in God (or Allah)
(2) worship five times daily, facing toward Mecca
(3) give alms or charity to those in need
(4) fast during the ninth month of the Muslim year
(5) make a pilgrimage to Mecca at least once during one's lifetime.

Muslims are also urged to refrain from drinking wine, touching or eating pork, gambling, usury (lending money at an excessive rate of interest), fraud, slander, and the making of images (Sachedina 2004). Muslims believe that life is a gift of God and the human body is given to serve God. Therefore, human life is respected and suicide, homicide and torture of the body in any form is prohibited.

One additional way to classify theories of ethics is to consider them consequential or nonconsequential. Consequential theories are those theories that look at the consequences of acts. They claim that an action is right to the extent that it produces good consequences and wrong to the extent that it produces bad consequences. Utilitarianism (Figure 2.1) is an example of a consequential ethical theory because it claims that an action is right if it tends to produce the greatest balance of value over disvalue (Beauchamp & Childress 2001). If an action does not do this, it is considered to be wrong.

Nonconsequential theories, on the other hand, are those theories that maintain that certain acts are right and others are wrong because they have or do not have right-making characteristics. Deontology is a type of nonconsequential theory that considers actions to be right based on laws or rules regarding duties or obligations (such as keeping promises, telling the truth, etc.) independent of their consequences or outcomes (Fry & Veatch 2006). One of the most prominent forms of deontology is Kant's theory of ethics (Figure 2.1), which holds that an action is right if it is done from duty and can be willed to be universal law for everyone (Kant 1964).

Principles of ethics

Traditional theories of ethics contain one or more ethical principles. Ethical principles are guides to moral decision making and moral action, and centre on the formation of moral judgments in professional practice (Beauchamp & Childress 2001). They generally assert that actions of a certain kind ought (or ought not) to be performed and serve to justify the rules that are often followed in patient care. The importance of applying ethical principles and rules in healthcare is increasingly recognised throughout the world. However, the way in which these principles are applied in a given situation within a specific culture may differ. For example, in most cultures, it is believed that the nurse should not lie to patients (agreement on the principle of veracity). Some behaviours would clearly be defined as lying in one country but would not be defined as lying in another. What constitutes a lie may differ between two countries so the principle might be applied differently in each country.

The ethical principles important to nursing practice are: beneficence and nonmaleficence, justice, autonomy, veracity and fidelity (Fry & Veatch 2006; Johnstone 2004).

Beneficence and nonmaleficence

Two key principles underpinning ethical practice in nursing and healthcare are those of beneficence (the obligation to do good) and nonmaleficence (the obligation to avoid doing harm) (Beauchamp & Childress 2001; Frankena 1973). Although obviously related, these principles are nevertheless distinct and it is important to recognise this distinction when used to guide moral conduct.

Acting on these principles can mean either helping others gain what is beneficial to them (e.g. that which actively promotes their welfare and well-being), and/or engaging in behaviours that will either prevent or reduce risks of harm to patients (e.g. that which could cause physical or psychological injury to patients, or deliberately violate their significant moral interests).

Applying these principles in nursing practice often poses difficult problems for the nurse. For example, it is not always clear if the nurse is obliged to consider all the ways in which the patient might be benefited or prevented from suffering a foreseeable harm. If nurses are obliged 'to promote health,' to prevent illness, to restore health and to alleviate suffering' (ICN 2006, p. 1), this is a substantial and complex amount of benefit for nurses to provide and may require very well developed skills – both professional and moral. If interpreted literally, it could entail many obligations toward the patient, some of which may be outside the expertise and resources of many nurses.

A second problem in applying these principles is deciding whether the obligation to provide benefit (beneficence) takes priority over the obligation to avoid harm (nonmaleficence). Some ethicists claim that the duty to avoid harm is actually a stronger obligation in healthcare relationships than the obligation to benefit (Beauchamp & Childress 2001; Ross 1939). This is because the resources needed to bestow a benefit might not be available, thus making it impossible for a person to fulfil his or her duty of beneficence – a failure which, ironically, could be construed as an unethical act. Avoiding causing deliberate harm and injury to others, however, is something that is within our individual capacity and resources. Any failure to uphold this principle, therefore, can be interpreted as a grossly unethical act regardless of the context. It is in this regard that the duty of nonmaleficence is sometimes seen to be stronger than the duty of beneficence.

Nonmaleficence as an action guiding principle of conduct has considerable importance in healthcare contexts. For example, physicians have often been urged 'above all [or first of all], do no harm' – primum non nocere – as part of the Hippocratic tradition in medical practice (Veatch 2000). Are nurses expected to follow a similar obligation to avoid harm more than provide benefit? This does not seem to be the case. In nursing, as is the case in other professional domains, the avoidance of harm is balanced by the provision of benefit, with acceptable ranges of both benefits and risks of harm established by standards of nursing practice and professional codes of ethics.

A third problem in applying this principle in nursing practice concerns the limits of providing benefits to patients. At what point do benefits to others (one's own family, the employing institution, co-workers) take priority over the potential benefits that the nurse might provide to the patient? Is the nurse obliged to provide benefits to anyone who might profit from nursing care and attention, or simply to the identified patient? Nurses need to be very clear about the boundaries of their obligation to provide benefits and avoid harms in patient care.

Justice

Once the boundaries of the obligation to provide benefit (beneficence) and avoid harm (nonmaleficence) are determined, nurses should be concerned about how benefits and burdens ought to be justly distributed among patient populations (Fry & Veatch 2006). In other words, the nurse must decide what is a just or fair allocation of healthcare resources and nursing care to patients under her care.

The principle of formal justice states that equals should be treated equally and that those who are unequal should be treated differently according to their needs (Beauchamp & Childress 2001). This means that those equal in health needs should receive the same amount of healthcare resources (equals should be treated equally). It also means that when some people have greater health needs than others, they should receive a greater amount of health resources (those who are unequal should be treated differently according to their needs). This type of allocation is just because it distributes health resources according to need in a fair (or ethical) manner.

Since it might not be possible to provide equal amounts of healthcare resources for all members of the society, policy should ensure that all individuals will have equal access to whatever healthcare resources are available, according to individual need. Once access to the healthcare system has been gained, however, people may be given different amounts of resources, depending on their needs. The focus on need allows for an ethical or fair distribution of available resources among patients and forgoes the distribution of these resources outside of need (Powers & Faden 2006).

Autonomy

The ethical principle of autonomy claims that individuals ought to be permitted personal liberty to determine their own actions according to plans that they have chosen (Beauchamp & Childress 2001; Fry & Veatch 2006). This means to respect individuals as self-determined choosers (Johnstone 2004). To respect persons as autonomous individuals is to acknowledge their choices which stem from personal values and beliefs.

One of the problems that arises in applying a principle of autonomy in nursing care is that patients often have varying capacities to be autonomous, depending on internal and external constraints. Internal constraints on patient autonomy are mental ability, level of consciousness, age and disease status. External constraints on patient autonomy often include the hospital environment, availability of nursing resources, the amount of information provided for making informed choices and the availability of financial resources.

The principle of autonomy may also be difficult to apply in patient care when the nurse or other members of the healthcare team believe that respecting the patient's choice is not in the best interests of the patient. In this type of situation, the nurse may need to consider the limits of individual patient autonomy and the criteria for justified paternalism. Paternalism is defined as the overriding of individual choices or intentional actions in order to provide benefit to that individual (Beauchamp & Childress 2001). Although paternalism is seldom justified in the care of patients, there is reason to believe that some situations warrant overriding patient autonomy when the benefits to be realised are great and the harms that will be avoided are significant (Beauchamp & Childress 2001).

Veracity

The principle of veracity is defined as the obligation to tell the truth and not to lie or deceive others. In many cultures, truthfulness has long been regarded as fundamental to the existence of trust among individuals. Because of this tradition, truthfulness enjoys a special significance in healthcare relationships in many parts of the world.

Truthfulness is generally expected as part of the respect that is owed persons (Fry & Veatch 2006). Individuals have the right to be told the truth and not to be lied to or deceived. Nurses are obliged to be truthful in culturally appropriate ways because not to do so may undermine the patient's trust and the overall therapeutic effectiveness of the nurse with the patient. In the long run, lack of truthfulness or its culturally inappropriate expression may bring about undesirable consequences for future relationships with patients and also for the patient's overall health and well-being (Johnstone 2004; Kanitsaki 1994).

In all cultures, truth-telling is a very complex task that must be handled in a culturally informed way. For example, some cultures highly value respecting patient autonomy and the rights of patients to know their medical diagnosis and prognosis. Thus, to withhold information about their medical diagnosis or prognosis from patients is generally regarded as being paternalistic and unjust. In other cultures, however, the patient is presumed to have a right not to know. Key to respecting patient autonomy in some cultural settings is respecting that the family has a legitimate and significant lay therapeutic role to play in imparting information to a sick loved one. In these cultures, it is common for family members to decide what information their loved one should be given, when, where, how and by whom (Johnstone 2004; Kanitsaki 1994). They will also ensure that any information that is given is imparted in a manner that will not undermine the patient's hope.

Fidelity

The principle of fidelity is defined as the obligation to remain faithful to one's commitments (Fry & Veatch 2006). Commitments that usually fall within the scope of fidelity are obligations implicit in a trusting relationship between patient and nurse, such as keeping promises and maintaining confidentiality.

Individuals tend to expect that promises will be kept in human relationships, and will not be broken without good reason. They have the same expectations concerning the obligation of confidentiality which is one of the most basic requirements of professional healthcare ethics. However, exceptions to both obligations can sometimes be made. For example, some individuals maintain that it is morally acceptable to break promises when the breaking of the promise produces more good than if the promise is kept. Confidences are often broken for the same reason. It is also generally accepted in moral philosophy that people are not bound to keep promises that commit them to doing something that is wrong or evil.

It is also argued that breaking promises and confidences is morally acceptable when the welfare of a third party is jeopardised by the keeping of the promise or confidence. An example of this situation is when presumed patient confidentiality is broken in order to report child abuse (Johnstone 2004) or the laboratory results of a serious communicable disease to a public health authority (Johnstone & Crock 1999). The information is reported only to the public health authority and to no one else, in order to protect the child from injury or to protect unsuspecting individuals from exposure to disease.

Others, however, argue against the breaking of confidences, particularly on the basis of benefits to other parties. They claim that keeping information confidential is a right-making characteristic, independent of consequences to others. While there may be good moral reasons to break promises to provide benefit to others, following the rule of not breaking confidences may be more ethical than merely providing the benefit.

One way to understand the conceptual nature of the moral commitments surrounding confidentiality and promise-keeping is to ground these obligations within an independent principle of fidelity (Fry & Veatch 2006). Thus, in order to be faithful in one's commitment to the patient, the nurse should carefully consider the information that should be kept confidential and what the nurse can reasonably agree to keep confidential. The nurse should also consider when promise-keeping is a legitimate expectation in the nurse–patient relationship and when it is not. One makes a commitment to keep confidentiality and keep promises only under conditions where it is possible to make such commitments. The duty to keep one's commitments in certain circumstances thus becomes the focus of these obligations and not just the general practice of keeping promises or confidentiality.

Beyond traditional theories of ethics and principlism

Traditional ethics has had a powerful influence on our understanding of the relevance of ethics to nursing practice. The forms of ethical discourse (descriptive, normative, metaethical), the methods of ethics (appeals to authority, consensus, intuition and the dialectic approach), theories of ethics and traditional principles of ethics influence the way we apply ethics in nursing practice. Traditional ethics is often criticised, however, for its limitations in healthcare practices, especially in relationships such as the nurse–patient relationship. Several philosophers (Blum 1994; Blustein 1991; MacIntyre 1985; Williams 1985) have criticised traditional ethical theory for its lack of attention to human emotions, to the roles of suffering and compassion and to the separation of ethical thought from the cultural, historical and social environments within which such thought occurs. Others have criticised principlism or the principle-oriented approach to healthcare ethics, because it relies on the structure of moral justification for ethical validity rather than the context within which ethical questions arise and decision making takes place (Clouser & Gert 1990; DeGrazia 1992; Toulmin 1981). For these reasons, many nursing leaders are considering other theories and approaches to ethics in order to understand ethical judgments and actions in nursing practice. Some are exploring the nature of morality and individuals' moral behaviours, especially the development of moral judgment in order to influence the moral development of nurse students during the nursing education process (Duckett & Ryden 1994).

Critique of principlism

Criticisms of traditional ethical theory seem to centre on the application of ethical principles (Clouser & Gert 1990) and the use of reason to determine what one ought to do (Kittay & Meyers 1987). In traditional ethical theories, people gain autonomy by using reason to discern which principles ought to be followed. By gaining personal autonomy in moral decision making, people also move toward their vision of the good. What is good is being able to make self-determined choices about one's life. By following rationally determined criteria for ethical reasoning, a person is a moral agent, capable of assuming responsibility for his or her moral deliberations. Individuals thus become self-governing, i.e. they not only become the source of the moral principles that they obey in their life, but are also subject to these principles in living their life.

This type of ethical deliberation considers moral agents to be individuals who are detached from the ethical situations in which they are involved. According to this view, ethical decision making involves an impersonal and impartial process that uses ethical principles and rules as absolute standards. The purpose of ethical decision making is to judge actions as right or wrong and apply principles to situations in an impartial manner. This is sometimes referred to as an 'ethic of strangers' rather than an 'ethic of intimates'. This ethic does not consider the importance of personal relationships between parties, but applies ethical principles impartially to the situation in much the same way as they have been applied in previous situations. The relationships involved in the current situation bear little or no relevance to the way in which principles are applied. Hence it is an ethic of strangers rather than an ethic of intimates, i.e. an ethic of people who have relationships with one another and a shared history.

The works of social psychologists Jean Piaget (1965) and Lawrence Kohlberg (1976, 1981) support this view of an ethics of strangers. Kohlberg, in particular, maintained that moral development involves a process whereby a person undergoes ever closer approximations to the traditional ethics ideal of a self-governing individual (1981). For him, the core of morality is justice. Other theorists, however, have not been willing to adopt this view of moral development and its association with traditional ethical theory and the principle-oriented approach to morality and moral judgment (Johnstone 1999).

James Rest, for example, argued that there is more to moral development than the development of moral judgment (Rest 1984). According to him, moral

Moral sensitivity	An awareness of how our actions affect other people. It involves being aware of different possible lines of action and how each line of action could affect the parties concerned. It involves imaginatively constructing possible scenarios, and knowing cause–consequence chains of events in the real world. It involves empathy and role-taking skills.
Moral judgment	Once the person is aware of possible lines of action and how people would be affected by each line of action (Component 1), then Component 2 judges which line of action is more morally justifiable (which alternative is just, or right).
Moral motivation	Concerns the importance given to moral values in competition with other values. Deficiencies in Component 1 occur when a person is not sufficiently motivated to put moral values higher than other values.
Moral character	Involves ego strength, perseverance, backbone, toughness, strength of conviction and courage. A person may be morally sensitive, may make good moral judgments, and may place high priority on moral values, but if the person wilts under pressure, is easily distracted or discouraged, is weak-willed, then moral failure occurs because of deficiency in Component 4, Interpersonal effectiveness and problem-solving skills are intimately connected to Component 4 processes.

Figure 2.3   The components of morality (Rest 1984, pp. 24–40).

behaviour is the end product of four distinct psychological processes: moral sensitivity, moral judgment, moral motivation and moral character (Figure 2.3). *Moral sensitivity* is the awareness of how our actions affect other people. It involves being aware of different possible actions and how each action could affect the parties concerned. *Moral judgment* concerns judging which action is more morally just or right (or morally justifiable) than other actions. *Moral motivation* involves the importance a person gives to moral values in competition with other values in making moral judgments. *Moral character* involves ego strength, perseverance, backbone, toughness, strength of conviction, and courage. A certain amount of each of psychological roughness and strong character is necessary to carry out moral action. If a deficiency occurs in any of these components, moral failure may result. Called the *Four-Component Model of Morality*, Rest contends that the four components comprise a logical analysis of what it takes to behave morally (Rest 1994).

Other approaches to ethics

Virtue-based theory (character ethics) focuses on the persons who perform actions and make various choices (Beauchamp & Childress 2001). Moral virtue is considered a character trait that is morally valued and that stems from the motivation to do what is right or good. Examples of moral virtues include courage, generosity, compassion, faithfulness and sincerity.

Rights-based theory emphasises the rights and obligations of persons in relation to one another. A right is a justified claim that can be made against an individual or groups. Having a right means that one can make moral demands on others or insist that one is due something. Legal rights are justified by legal principles and rules; moral rights are justified by moral principles and rules. Examples of rights common to Western ethics include the right to life, health, healthcare, abortion and self-determination.

Community-based theory (communitarianism) emphasises the common good, communal values, social goals and tradition as the foundations for ethical judgments (Beauchamp & Childress 2001). It rejects the liberalism of utilitarianism and the individualism that characterises Kant's theory of ethics. Instead, it embraces communal values, such as family cohesion, equality, privacy and ideas about the social good (Gross 1999). Communitarism often provides the basis for organ donation regulations and healthcare delivery systems of care.

Relationship-based theory emphasises 'traits valued in intimate personal relationships, such as sympathy, compassion, fidelity, discernment and love' (Beauchamp & Childress 2001, p. 369). One type of relationship-based theory focuses on an ethic of care where caring is viewed as a behaviour, or set of behaviours, that stems from a strong opinion, feeling, concern or interest in something or someone and contributes to the good, worth, dignity or comfort of someone (Fry 2004a; Fry, Killen & Robinson 1996). Some view an ethic of care as a type of virtue theory (Noddings 1984) while others view it as a moral-point-of-view theory (Blustein 1991). Regardless of its form, an ethic of care is an alternative normative ethical theory for deciding what is right and wrong, good or bad, or obligatory in human relationships.

Another type of relationship-based theory focuses on relational ethics where the quality of relationships between the nurse and his or her patients or colleagues needs as much attention as the quality of clinical competence (Bergum 2004). Relational ethics is concerned with the kinds of relationships that allow for 'the flourishing of good rather than evil, trust rather than fear, difference rather than sameness, healing rather than surviving' (p. 487). A key element in this approach to ethics is trust in colleagues' expertise, knowledge, and being available to each other (Rodney, Brown & Liaschenko 2004). Ethics is thus concerned with the quality of every situation, every encounter, and with every patient. Each nurse is morally responsible for personal actions in relation to the people he or she cares for, educates, supervises, or works with in partnership (Lindh, Severinsson & Berg 2007).

Support for an ethic of care

One of Kohlberg's students, Carol Gilligan (1982), conducted her own research on the moral development of women and their decision-making strategies. Her research suggests that the principle-oriented approach to ethics does not reflect the kind of ethical concerns confronting women or how women make ethical decisions in their lives. She also questioned whether Kohlberg's theory adequately reflected the course of moral development in women. Her research shows that rather than applying abstract ethical principles to moral issues according

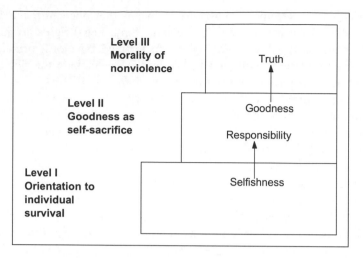

Figure 2.4   Carol Gilligan's model of moral development (1982).

to traditional theories of ethics, women employ different strategies in making moral decisions. Their strategies centre on the nature of care and responsibility in relationships and aim at maintaining ties with individuals and maintaining self-integrity. Her research participants did not describe conflicts of rights as ethical problems. Instead, ethical problems resulted from the contextual nature of individual relationships, and the perceived obligations within relationships.

Gilligan's research also indicates that the moral development of women is different from that of men and equally worthy. She describes three levels of development, each with two transitional stages, that involve consideration of care and responsibility in a woman's relationships with others (Figure 2.4). Progressive moral development leads to the maintenance of personal integrity and care for oneself without neglecting others with whom one has relationships. While Kohlberg's theory of moral development is supported by the well-known and established rationalist system of ethical theorising, Gilligan's theory of moral development is supported by references to Aristotle's ethics with its focus on moral character (Aristotle 1962) and philosopher David Hume's ethics grounded in emotion and personal concern (Hume 1978). Hume, in particular, doubted that reason could move an individual to act morally. For him, ethical life is guided by moral sentiments and obligations to the relationships that one has with others.

Building on Gilligan's theory of moral development in women, philosopher Nel Noddings (1984) proposed an ethic of care theory complete with notions about moral obligation, moral good and moral justification. Noddings views the ethic of care as a type of virtue theory where moral ideals are preferable to ethical principles as guides to moral action. Noddings centres her ideas on the value of care and the attitude of caring which expresses our earliest memories of being cared for by someone else. Caring involves behaviours that have moral content and that can be adopted by both men and women. To care is to be 'charged with the protection, welfare, or maintenance of something or someone' (Noddings 1984, p. 2). Ethical caring involves a relationship where one meets another morally. Motivated by the ideal of caring where we join with others as partners in human relationships, 'we are guided not by ethical principles', states Noddings, 'but by the strength of the ideal of caring itself'. Rather than the conditions for moral justification that permeate traditional theories of ethics, the ethic of care simply depends on 'the maintenance of conditions that will permit caring to flourish' (Noddings 1984, p. 5).

A theory of nursing ethics

It is not clear that a theory of ethics unique to nursing can be described or is even necessary (Volker 2003). However, if a theory of nursing ethics can be described, it needs to have several characteristics. First, it should have a focus on human well-being as its central moral good (Fry 2004b). Nursing is, after all, a practice that seeks human well-being by promoting health, preventing illness, restoring health and alleviating suffering (ICN 2006). Nurses have a primary professional responsibility to people who require nursing care and are obliged to promote their well-being, regardless of their health status.

Second, a theory of nursing ethics should emphasise caring as a moral obligation. Several nurse theorists have already declared caring to be a central value for the ethical dimensions of nursing practice (Gadow 1985; Tschudin 1992). Gadow (1985), for example, argues that the value of caring supports a nursing ethic that will protect and enhance the human dignity of patients receiving healthcare. She views caring in the nurse–patient relationship as a commitment to certain ends for the patient, and analyses caring as demonstrated in the nursing actions of truth-telling and touch.

Others have considered caring as central to nursing as a moral practice (Bishop & Scudder 1990; Gastmans, Dierckz deCasterle & Schotsmans 1998). These views assert that there is a caring relationship as a condition for nursing practice, caring behaviours that comprise nursing activities and a goal of 'good' care as a result of nursing activities. Care is not just a foundation for nursing practice but is essential to the excellence of that practice. Good care thus includes attention to the physical, relational, social, psychological, moral and spiritual dimensions of the patient's care as central components in the nurse–patient relationship.

Others have promoted caring as a way of knowing and not knowing (Benner 1991, 1994) and as the necessary basis for nurses' ethical judgments (Nortvedt 1996). Still others, however, criticise the care perspective as a basis for nurses' ethical judgments because (1) it rejects ethical principles and promotes a mode of moral reasoning based on relationships (Rudnick 2001); (2) it emphasises the caring relationship between nursing and patient rather than the individuals in that relationship (Tarlier 2004; Warelow 1996); and (3) the caring ideal is a vice rather than a virtue in that it promotes dependency, sexism, unfairness, emotional attachment and burnout (Curzer 1993). Despite these criticisms, caring is still considered essential to ethical nursing practice.

Third, a theory of nursing ethics should emphasise the importance of moral character in the nurse–patient relationship (Armstrong 2006; Begley 2006). It will be, in part, a virtue theory where nurses are motivated to do good acts that promote patient well-being. A nurse who is a morally good person will have the desires and motives to promote patient well-being (Barker 2000; Tuckett 1998). Such a nurse will be more likely to understand what should be done in the nursing role, more likely to perform the actions that are required and more likely to act on moral ideals (Arries 2005; Beauchamp & Childress 2001; Pullman 1994).

Fourth, a theory of nursing ethics should set aside the notion that ethical principles and rules have a primary role to play in providing moral justification for nurses' judgments and actions. Studies of ethical decision-making frameworks used by nurses have found both principle-oriented and care-oriented approaches (Cooper 1991; Parker 1990; Redman & Fry 2000). Likewise, studies of moral sensitivity and moral reasoning among health professionals have found that most professionals use both care-oriented and principle-oriented approaches (Bebeau & Brabeck 1989). The results of these studies support the notion that nurses integrate theoretical approaches to ethics in their ethical decision making. These approaches include notions of moral good, moral obligation, character ethics and principlism (Rodney, Varcoe, Storch, McPherson, Mahoney, Brown, Pauly, Hartrick & Starzomski 2002). Principles guide decisions related to the just allocation of healthcare resources (Emanuel 2000) and are firmly anchored in contemporary bioethics thought (Evans 2000). Nurses emphasise an approach, depending on which aspects of an event they are involved with (Bebeau & Brabeck 1989; Smith & Godfrey 2002). Thus, a theory of nursing ethics will include ethical principles so that nurses can use them in justifying ethical decisions in nursing practice (Johnstone 2004).

Ethics and the law

Legal questions often play a prominent role in the consideration of ethical issues. This is not surprising since legal and ethical standards often develop within the same historical, social, cultural and philosophical climates. Yet the significant differences between ethics and the law are important to recognise. Many nursing actions may be both legal and ethical while others may be legal, but not ethical, or ethical, but not legal. In some countries, it may be considered both legal and ethical for a nurse to participate in an abortion. In other countries, it would be illegal to participate in any abortion even though the individual nurse may believe the abortion to be ethically justified (for example, if the woman had been raped or the pregnancy was endangering the life of the mother). Yet even in countries where abortion is legally obtained, many individuals consider it unethical to participate in the procedure due to deeply held religious beliefs and values.

One reason that ethics and the law are often confused is that both law and ethics use the term 'rights'. Individuals have legal rights (i.e. innocent until proven guilty) which are grounded in the law; they also have moral rights (i.e. right to life) which are grounded in ethical systems, principles and rules. Legal rights are claims recognised as valid by the legal system while moral rights are usually derived from theoretical considerations of customs, traditions and ideals and are not necessarily upheld by legal rules. In protecting or defending certain rights of the patient, nurses may be uncertain whether legal standards or ethical standards will justify their actions. Many moral rights of patients (i.e. self-determination) may be protected by law (informed consent to treatment, for example) but this is not always the case. A patient may claim a moral right to die and not be kept alive by a ventilator or by artificially supplied nutrition and hydration when suffering from the end-stage of a serious illness or incompetent or irreversibly comatose. Yet disconnecting a patient from a ventilator or withdrawing nutrition and hydration from him under these conditions may be illegal for the health professional, bearing in mind that the legality of such actions may vary from legal jurisdiction to jurisdiction and country to country (Johnstone 1996).

Codes of nursing ethics may also be protected by law when professional nursing associations convince their governments to recognise and regulate professional nursing by legislation. In those countries where the government has translated the basic principles of the nursing code of ethics into enforceable rules of law, it is possible to consider the legal implications of following or not following the professional code of ethics. We may learn a lot about ethics by studying and criticising the law because legal cases often contain a great deal of ethical reasoning. However, the law only provides a background against which we reflect upon, consider and make ethical decisions. Nurses need to use their knowledge of ethics and ethical reasoning to make ethical decisions while using their knowledge of the law to determine the legal parameters of nursing practice (Johnstone 1994). Nurses also need to keep ethics and the law separate because without this distinction it would not be possible to find a position from which to criticise and reject law that, while valid, is nevertheless morally bad.

Bioethics

Following World War II, medical and scientific technology developed and expanded at tremendous speed, giving the medical profession increasing control over disease and death. It also created unprecedented moral questions about how and when technology ought to be used to keep people alive, to treat otherwise fatal disorders, to conduct experimental research and even to alter the human genome. As technological advances make it possible to dramatically alter life, death and the human condition, questions arise that require new types of legal and moral responses and decisions. Bioethics (from the Greek *bios*, meaning life, literally ethics in the bio-realm or 'life ethics'), or applied ethics in the biomedical sciences, is a relatively new mode of inquiry within the discipline of ethics that attempts to provide moral responses to these difficult questions (Jecker, Jonsen & Pearlman 2007; Jonsen 1998; Reich 1995).

During its first stage of development, bioethics focused on medical ethics, the ethical norms for the practice of medicine. The development of professional codes of medical ethics, the influences of secular and nonsecular ethical traditions on medical ethics and the Hippocratic tradition were the central themes of this stage of bioethics. Some early scholars in medical ethics claimed that all applications of ethics to problems in the medical sphere are part of medical ethics (Veatch 2000). Physician ethics, nurse ethics, social work ethics, dentist ethics and chaplain ethics were regarded as branches of medical ethics. Later, however, it was recognised that some of these so-called branches of medical ethics are substantially different from one another and from medical ethics. As a result, medical ethics is no longer considered the major content area of bioethics.

The second stage of development in bioethics occurred along with the growth of new knowledge through systematic human experimentation. The development of codes of research ethics, regulations for the protection of human subjects in research, and the social and moral consequences of research have been central themes of this stage (Council of Europe 1997; National Commission 1978; Schmidt 2000; Wachter 1997). Specific contributions of bioethics to research ethics are discussed in detail in Chapter 12.

The third stage of development in bioethics has been marked by efforts to formulate public policy guidelines for clinical care, allocation of healthcare resources and patient access to healthcare services. Governments have designated various groups to study these problems and formulate recommendations (Council of Europe 1997; President's Commission 1983). For example, the President's Commission for the Study of Ethical Problems in Medicine and Biomedical and Behavioral Research (1983) issued public reports and recommendations on ethical topics such as the definition of death, forgoing life-sustaining treatment, genetic counselling and research, informed consent and access to healthcare, to name a few. Private organisations have also assembled working groups to establish guidelines for healthcare delivery (Smith 1999).

Throughout its development, bioethics has relied on traditional areas of ethical inquiry, appealing to traditional methods of argumentation in applying ethical reasoning to complex moral questions.

Summary

Ethics is a discipline that provides theoretical approaches for ethical decision making and action. The types of subject matter of ethics, the methods of argumentation typically used in ethical discourse, and the ethical principles and rules contained in various ethical theories stem from a rich historical and philosophical tradition. The practice of nursing requires familiarity with both traditional and contemporary forms of ethical theorising. Contemporary ethical thought does not have quite the rich tradition that rationalist approaches to ethics have enjoyed; however, it does have strong roots in Aristotelian ethics and other ethical systems of thought. In addition, nurses should be able to apply traditional ethical principles in nursing practice along with the contextual consideration of the ethic of care and responsibility in human relationships. The practice of nursing will be enriched when both approaches are used in resolving ethical questions related to patient care. The nurse is advised to follow ethical standards for making ethical decisions and to follow legal standards for determining the legal dimensions of nursing practice. As nurses incorporate knowledge of ethics into their approaches to patient care, they will contribute to the growth of bioethics as a discipline, and function more effectively as moral agents in the healthcare system of their country.

References

Aristotle (1962) *Nicomachean ethics*. Trans by M. Ostwald. Indianapolis: Bobbs-Merrill.

Armstrong, A.E. (2006) Towards a strong virtue ethics for nursing practice. *Nurs Philos* 7(3), 110–124.

Arries, E. (2005) Virtue ethics: An approach to moral dilemmas in nursing. *Curationis* 28(3), 64–72.

Barker, P. (2000) Reflections on caring as a virtue ethic within an evidence-based culture. *Int J Nurs Studies* 37, 329–336.

Beauchamp, T.L. & Childress, J.F. (2001) *Principles of biomedical ethics*, 5th ed. New York: Oxford University Press.

Bebeau, M.J. & Brabeck, M. (1989) Ethical sensitivity and moral reasoning among men and women in the professions. In M.M. Brabeck (Ed) *Who cares?: Theory, research, and educational implications of the ethic of care* (pp. 144–163). New York: Praeger.

Begley, A.M. (2006) Facilitating the development of moral insight in practice: Teaching ethics and teaching virtue. *Nurs Philos* 7(4), 257–265.

Benner, P. (1991) The role of experience, narrative, and community in skilled ethical comportment. *Advances in Nursing Science* 14(2), 1–21.

Benner, P. (Ed.) (1994) *Interpretive phenomenology: Embodiment, caring, and ethics in health and illness*. Thousand Oaks, CA: Sage.

Bergum, V. (2004) Relational ethics in nursing. In J.L. Storch, P. Rodney & R. Starzomski (Eds) *Toward a moral horizon: Nursing ethics for leadership and practice* (pp. 485–503). Toronto: Pearson, Prentice Hall.

Bishop, A.H. & Scudder, J. (1990) *The practical, moral and personal sense of nursing: A phenomenological philosophy of practice*. Albany, NY: State University of New York Press.

Blum, L.A. (1994) *Moral perception and particularity*. New York: Cambridge University Press.

Blustein, J. (1991) *Care and commitment: Taking the personal point of view*. New York: Oxford University Press.

Clouser, K.D. & Gert, B. (1990) A critique of principlism. *J Med & Philosophy* 15, 219–236.

Cooper, M.C. (1991) Principle-oriented ethics and the ethic of care: A creative tension. *ANS* 14(2), 22–31.

Council of Europe (1997) *Convention for the protection of human rights and dignity of the human being with regard to the application of biology and medicine: Convention on human rights and biomedicine*. European Treaty Series No. 164.

Coward, H., Lipner, J. & Young, K. (1989) *Hindu ethics: Purity, abortion, and euthanasia*. Albany: State University of New York Press.

Curzer, H. (1993) Is care a virtue for health care professionals? *Journal of Medicine and Philosophy* 18(1), 51–69.

Damasio, A. (1994) *Descartes' error: Emotion, reason, and the human brain*. New York: Avon Books.

Davis-Floyd, R. & Arvidson, P. Sven (Eds) (1997) *Intuition: The inside story*. New York: Routledge.

DeGrazia, D. (1992) Moving forward in bioethical theory: Theories, cases, and specified principlism. *J. Med & Philosophy* 17, 511–539.

Duckett, L.J. & Ryden, M.B. (1994) Education for ethical nursing practice. In J.R. Rest & D. Narvaez (Eds) *Moral development in the professions: psychology and applied ethics* (pp. 51–70). Hillsdale, NJ: Lawrence Erlbaum Associates.

Emanuel, E.J. (2000) Justice and managed care: Four principles for the just allocation of health care resources. *Hast Ctr Rprt* 30(3), 8–16.

Evans, J.H. (2000) A sociological account of the growth of principlism. *Hast Ctr Rprt* 30(5), 31–38.

Frankena, W.K. (1973) *Ethics*, 2nd. ed. Englewood Cliffs, NJ: Prentice-Hall.

Fry, S.T. (1992) Neglect of philosophical inquiry in nursing: Cause and effect. In J.F. Kikuchi & H. Simmons (Eds) *Philosophic inquiry in nursing* (pp. 85–96). Newbury Park, CA: Sage Publications.

Fry, S.T. (2004a) Nursing ethics. In G. Khushf (Ed) *Handbook of bioethics: Taking stock of the field from a philosophical perspective* (pp. 489–505). New York: Kluwer Academic Publishers.

Fry, S.T. (2004b) Nursing ethics. In S.G. Post (Ed) *Encyclopedia of bioethics*, 3rd ed (1898–1903). New York: Macmillan Reference USA: Thomson/Gale.

Fry, S.T. (1989) Toward a theory of nursing ethics. *ANS* 11(4), 9–22.

Fry, S.T., Killen, A.R. & Robinson, E.M. (1996) Care-based reasoning, caring, and the ethic of care: A need for clarity. *J Clin Ethics* 7(1), 41–47.

Fry, S.T. & Veatch, R.M. (2006) *Case studies in nursing ethics*, 3rd ed. Boston: Jones & Bartlett.

Gadow, S. (1985) Nurse and patient: The caring relationship. In A.H. Bishop & J.R. Scudder (Eds) *Caring, curing, coping: Nurse, physician, patient relationships* (pp. 31–43). Birmingham, AL: University of Alabama Press.

Gastmans, D., Dierckx deCasterle, B. & Schotsmans, P. (1998) Nursing considered as moral practice: A philosophical–ethical interpretation of nursing. *KIEJ* 8(1), 43–69.

Gilligan, C. (1982) *In a different voice*. Cambridge, MA: Harvard University Press.

Griffin, A.P. (1983) A philosophical analysis of caring in nursing. *J Adv Nurs* 8, 289–295.

Gross, M.L. (1999) Autonomy and paternalism in communitarian society: Patient rights in Israel. *Hast Ctr Rprt* 29(4), 13–20.

Harvey, P. (2000) *An introduction to Buddhist ethics: Foundation, values, and issues*. New York: Cambridge University Press.

Hume, D. (1978) *A treatise of human nature*. L.A. Selby-Bigge & P.H. Nidditch (Eds). Oxford: Clarendon Press.

International Council of Nurses (2006) *Code of ethics for nurses*. Geneva: International Council of Nurses.

Jecker, N., Jonsen, A. & Pearlman, R. (2007) *Bioethics: an introduction to the history, methods and practice*, 2nd ed. Sudbury, MA: Jones & Bartlett.

Johnstone, M.-J. (1994) *Nursing and the injustices of the law*. Sydney: WB Saunders/ Baillière Tindall.

Johnstone, M.-J. (Ed) (1996) *The politics of euthanasia: A nursing response*. Canberra: Royal College of Nursing, Australia.

Johnstone, M.-J. (1998) *Determining and responding effectively to ethical professional misconduct: A report to the Nurses Board of Victoria*. Melbourne.

Johnstone, M.-J. (1999) *Bioethics: A nursing perspective*, 3rd ed. Sydney: Harcourt Saunders.

Johnstone, M.-J. (2004) *Bioethics: A nursing perspective*, 4th ed. Sydney: Elsevier Australia.

Johnstone, M.-J. & Crock, E. (1999) Nurses with blood-borne pathogens and the moral responsibilities of nurse regulating authorities. *Australian Journal of Advanced Nursing*, 16(3): 7–13.

Jonsen, A.R. (1998) *The birth of bioethics*. New York: Oxford University Press.

Kanitsaki, O. (1994) Cultural and linguistic diversity. In J. Romanini and J. Daly (Eds) *Critical care nursing: Australian perspective* (pp. 94–125). Sydney: Baillière Tindall/ W.B. Saunders.

Kant, I. (1964) *Groundwork of the metaphysics of morals*. Trans. by H.J. Paton. New York: Harper & Row.

Ketefian, S. & Fry, S.T. (1998) Research in nursing ethics. In J. Fitzpatrick (Ed) *Encyclopedia of nursing research* (pp. 493–495). New York: Springer.

King, L. & Clark, J.M. (2002) Intuition and the development of expertise in surgical ward and intensive care nurses. *J Adv Nurs* 37(4), 322–329.

Kittay, E.F. & Meyers, D.T. (Eds) (1987) *Women and moral theory*. Totowa, NJ: Rowman & Littlefield.

Kohlberg, L. (1976) Moral stages and moralization: The cognitive–developmental approach. In T. Lickona (Ed) *Moral development and behavior: Theory, research and social issues* (pp. 31–53). New York: Holt, Rinehart and Winston.

Kohlberg, L. (1981) *The philosophy of moral development*. San Francisco, CA: Harper & Row.

Kopelman, L. (1995) Conceptual and moral disputes about futile and useful treatments. *J Med & Philosophy* 20(2), 109–121.

Ladd, J. (1978) The task of ethics. In W.T. Reich (Ed) *Encyclopedia of Bioethics* (pp. 400–407). New York: The Free Press.

Lindh, I. B., Severinsson, E. & Berg, A. (2007) Moral responsibility: A relational way of being. *Nurs Ethics* 14(2), 129–140.

MacIntyre, A. (1985) *After virtue: A study in moral theory*. Notre Dame: University of Notre Dame Press.

McCarthy, J. (2006) A pluralist view of nursing ethics. *Nurs Philos* 7(3), 157–164.

National Commission for the Protection of Human Subjects of Biomedical and Behavioral Research (1978) *The Belmont Report: Ethical Principles and Guidelines for the Protection of Human Subjects of Research.* Washington, DC: US Government Printing Office.

Nielsen, L. (1989) *Why be moral?* Buffalo, New York: Prometheus Books.

Noddings, N. (1984) *Caring: A feminine approach to ethics & moral education*. Berkeley: University of California Press.

Nortvedt, P. (1996) *Sensitive judgment: Nursing, moral philosophy, and an ethic of care.* Oslo, Norway: Tano Aschehoug.

Nyitay, V.L. (2004) Confucianism. In S.G. Post (Ed) *Encyclopedia of bioethics*, 3rd ed (pp. 508–513). New York: Macmillan Reference USA: Thomson/Gale.

Parker, R.S. (1990) Nurses' stories: The search for a relational ethic of care. *ANS* 13(1), 31–40.

Piaget, J. (1965) *The moral judgment of the child*. New York: The Free Press.

Powers, M. & Faden, R. (2006) *Social justice: the moral foundations of public health and health policy.* New York: Oxford University Press.

President's Commission for the Study of Ethical Problems in Medicine and Biomedical and Behavioral Research (1983) *Summary*. Washington, DC: US Government Printing Office.

Pullman, D. (1994) Can virtue be bought?: Moral education and the commodification of values. *Teaching Phil* 17(4), 321–333.

Redman, B.K. & Fry, S.T. (2000) Nurses' ethical conflicts: What is really known about them? *Nurs Ethics* 2(4), 360–366.

Reich, W. (1995) The word 'bioethics': the struggle over its earliest meanings. *KEIJ* 5(1), 19–34.

Rest, J. R. (1984) The major components of morality. In W. Kurtines & J. Gewirtz (Eds) *Morality, moral behavior, and moral development* (pp. 24–40). New York: Wiley.

Rest, J.R. (1994) Background: Theory and research. In J.R. Rest & D. Narvaez (Eds) *Moral development in the professions: Psychology and applied ethics* (pp. 1–26). Hillsdale, NJ: Lawrence Erlbaum Associates.

Rodney, P., Brown, H. & Liaschenko, F. (2004) Moral agency: Relational connections and trust. In J.L. Storch, P. Rodney & R. Starzomski (Eds) *Toward a moral horizon* (pp. 154–177). Toronto: Pearson, Prentice Hall.

Rodney, P., Varcoe, C., Storch, J.L., McPherson, G., Mahoney, K., Brown, H., Pauly, B., Hartrick, G. & Starzomski, R. (2002) Navigating towards a moral horizon: A multisite qualitative study of ethical practice in nursing. *Can J Nurs Res* 34(3), 75–102.

Ross, W.D. (1939) *The right and the good.* Oxford: Oxford University Press.

Rudnick, A. (2001) A meta-ethical critique of care ethics. *Theor Med Bioeth* 22(6), 505–517.

Sachedina, A. (2004) Islam, bioethics. In S.G. Post (Ed) *Encyclopedia of Bioethics*, 3rd ed (pp. 1330–1338). New York: Macmillan Reference USA: Thomson/Gale.

Saddhatissa, H. (1987) *Buddhist ethics: The path to Nirvana.* London, UK: Wisdom Publications.

Schmidt, K.W. (2000) The concealed and the revealed: Bioethical issues in Europe at the end of the second millennium. *J Med & Philosophy* 25(2), 123–132.

Smith, K.V. & Godfrey, N.S. (2002) Being a good nurse and doing the right thing: A qualitative study. *Nurs Ethics* 9(3), 301–312.

Smith, R. (1999) Shared ethical principles for everybody in health care: A working draft from the Tavistock Group. *BMJ* 318, 248–251.

Tarlier, D.S. (2004) Beyond caring: The moral and ethical bases of responsive nurse–patient relationships. *Nurs Philos* 5(3), 230–241.

Thompson, M. (2003) *Eastern philosophy.* London: Hodder Arnold.

Toulmin, S. (1981) The tyranny of principles. *Hast Ctr Rep* 11(6), 31–39.

Tschudin, V. (1992) *Ethics in nursing: The caring relationship*, 2nd ed. London: Butterworth Heinemann.

Tuckett, A. (1998) The virtues of nursing. *Kai Tiaki: Nurs N Zealand* August, 24–25.

Veatch, R.M. (2000) *The basics of bioethics.* Upper Saddle River, NJ: Prentice Hall.

Volker, D.L. (2003) Is there a unique nursing ethic? *Nurs Sci Q* 16(3), 207–211.

Wachter, M.A.M. (1997) The European Convention on Bioethics. *Hast Ctr Rprt* 27(1), 13–23.

Warelow, P.J. (1996) Is caring the ethical ideal? *Journal of Advanced Nursing* 24, 655–661.

Weiss, M.G. (2004) Hinduism. In S.G. Post (Ed) *Encyclopedia of Bioethics*, 3rd ed (pp. 1142–1149). New York: Macmillan Reference USA: Thomson/Gale.

Williams, B. (1985) *Ethics and the limits of philosophy.* Cambridge: Harvard University Press.

Chapter 3
Ethical concepts for nursing practice

Advocacy, accountability, cooperation and caring are among the ethical concepts that provide a foundation for nurses' ethical decision making. The concepts discussed here were selected to illustrate the ethical values and standards that have found expression in the nursing profession's rich and distinctive history as a morally accountable profession.

Advocacy

The ICN (2006) *Code of Ethics for Nurses* makes plain that the nurse's primary responsibility is to people who require nursing care (p. 2). Fulfilling this responsibility may sometimes require nurses to assume an 'advocacy role', for example, in situations where a person's entitlements to and in healthcare are being undermined in some way. Advocacy is widely recognised within the nursing ethics literature and nursing codes of ethics as a professional ideal and as a 'moral imperative' (Grace 2001; MacDonald 2006). If nurses are to be able to respond to this moral imperative effectively and fulfil their responsibilities as 'advocates' (whether in individual and immediate practice settings, or in broader social contexts) they need to have at least a working knowledge and understanding of the concept of advocacy and its possible role in the profession and practice of nursing (Grace 2001; MacDonald 2006)

Advocacy is commonly defined as 'an action that an advocate takes to represent the cause of another' (MacDonald 2006, p. 120). In a legal context, the term 'advocacy' refers to the role of a lawyer or legal counsellor to 'act solely and diligently in the interests of the client' (Grace 2001, p. 154). Moreover, while representing the client, the lawyer's *foremost responsibility is to the client.*

Advocacy, as a term, has its origins in law. Some contend that because the legal sense of the term has a very distinctive meaning and application in legal contexts, its translation and use in healthcare settings is problematic (Grace 2001). Nonetheless, many hospitals around the world have adopted the notion of

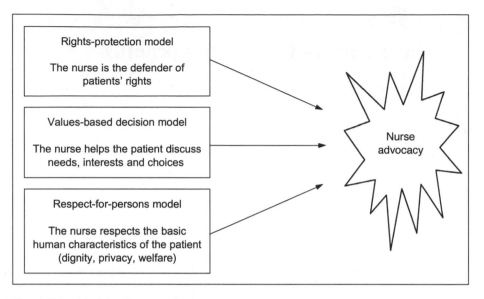

Figure 3.1   Models of nurse advocacy.

patient advocate and have employed 'patient advocates' (more commonly called 'patient representatives') to uphold and protect the rights of patients who, for various reasons, are either unable or unwilling to protect their own rights to and in healthcare. In keeping with this 'patients' rights' view of advocacy, the principal role of the patient advocate/patient representative in hospital contexts is to speak on the patient's behalf in much the same way as an attorney might plead the case of his or her client in a court of law.

The term 'advocacy' has also been used to describe the nature of the nurse–patient relationship. Several interpretations of advocacy in the literature describe this relationship in slightly different ways. One interpretation (and one that has prevailed in nursing contexts), is the patients' rights protection model (Figure 3.1). This model views the nurse as the 'defender' of patient rights within the healthcare system. The nurse informs patients of their rights, makes sure that the patients understand these rights, reports any infringements and acts to prevent any further infringements of the patient's bona fide rights claims. In summary, this interpretation views the nurse as an arbitrator for the patient's human rights to and in healthcare.

A second interpretation, values-based decision model (Figure 3.1), views the nurse as the person who helps the patient discuss his or her needs, interests and choices consistent with the patient's values and lifestyle. The nurse does not impose decisions or values on the patient but helps the patient examine the advantages and disadvantages of various health options in order to make decisions most consistent with his or her values and beliefs.

A third interpretation, respect-for-persons model (Figure 3.1), views the patient as a fellow human being entitled to respect. As advocate, the nurse first considers the basic human values of the patient and then acts to uphold and protect the patient's human dignity, privacy and choices. When the patient is incapable of making choices, the nurse advocates the patient's welfare as defined by the patient before he or she became ill or as defined by his or her family members or surrogate decision makers. If no one is available to define the welfare of the patient, the nurse promotes the best interests of the patient to the best of his or her nursing ability. The nurse assumes responsibility for the way in which the patient's significant human values are protected during his or her illness, being accountable to society and to the nursing profession for the way in which this important advocate role is carried out.

The foregoing model of advocacy is consistent with the values and moral imperatives expressed in a variety of nursing codes of ethics (MacDonald 2006), including the International Council of Nurses (ICN) *Code of Ethics for Nurses* (2006). The ICN Code, for example, prescribes that nurses have a responsibility to take 'appropriate action to safeguard individuals, families and communities when their health is endangered by a co-worker or any other person' (ICN 2006, p. 3). This prescription basically requires the nurse to *act* to protect individual patients, their families and/or significant others, and communities from harm. Actions taken in response to this moral imperative may have important long range implications for the safety and quality of patient care and the broader advocacy role of the nurse within the healthcare system and the community (Grace 2001; Jardin 2001; McMurray 1991).

Accountability/responsibility

The concept of accountability has two major attributes: answerability and responsibility (Fry 2004). Accountability can be defined as being answerable for one's actions, and entails giving satisfactory reasons and explanations for one's actions or how one has carried out one's responsibility (Fry-Revere 1992). Responsibility includes not only 'one's intentional conduct', but 'anything with which one is seen to have a causal relationship (whether this perception is justified or not)' (Fry-Revere 1992, p. 5).

In the ICN *Code of Ethics for Nurses* (2006), the responsibility of the nurse is to:

- promote health
- prevent illness
- restore health
- alleviate suffering

A nurse is accountable when he or she explains how this responsibility has been carried out, justifying the choices and actions in accordance with accepted principles and standards of professional nursing conduct and ethics.

Accountability is an important ethical concept because nursing practice involves a relationship between the nurse and the patient. As the noted American nurse theorist Virginia Henderson (1977) states in her classic work *Basic Principles of Nursing Care*:

'The unique function of the nurse is to assist the individual, sick or well, in the performance of those activities contributing to health or its recovery (or to peaceful death) that he would perform unaided if he had the necessary strength, will or knowledge' (p. 4).

Having agreed to provide nursing care, the nurse can be held accountable for providing such care according to principles and standards of ethical professional conduct. Nursing accountability even extends beyond the individual nurse–patient relationship to others who may not be nurses, and to employers (Johnstone 2001; Rowe 2000). The nurse may be accountable to the patient, the profession, the employer, and to society for what has been done (or not done) in providing nursing care. Public trust and confidence in the nursing profession may depend on its practitioners being seen as accountable and responsible (NMC 2004).

Legal accountability for nursing practice is specified by licensure or registration procedures and nurse practice acts/legislation. Moral accountability for nursing practice is specified in the ICN *Code of Ethics for Nurses* (2006) and other standards of nursing practice established by the members of the profession. In the American Nurses Association *Code of Ethics for Nurses* (2001), it is noted that accountability means 'to be answerable to oneself and others for one's own actions' (p. 16).

The United Kingdom Nursing and Midwifery Council's (NMC) *Code of Professional Conduct* (2004) states that 'As a registered nurse, midwife or specialist community public health nurse . . . you are personally accountable for your practice. This means that you are answerable for your actions and omissions, regardless of advice or directions from another professional' (Standard 1.3). The Canadian Nurses' Association (CNA) (2002) *Code of Ethics for Registered Nurses*, likewise states: 'Nurses are answerable for their practice, and they act in a manner consistent with their professional responsibilities and standards of practice' (p. 16). The Singapore Nursing Board (2006) states that nurses and midwives will 'provide care in a responsible and accountable manner' and that this includes alerting an appropriate authority 'of any situations which endanger the health and safety of clients or colleagues' (Value Statement 5). Similarly the Nursing Council of Hong Kong's *Code of Professional Conduct and Codes of Ethics* (1999) states: 'The nurse is responsible and accountable for individual nursing judgements and actions', and 'The nurse ensures that there is no action or omission of responsibility that is detrimental to the interests and safety of patients/clients' (Standards 4.2 & 4.3). The Australian Nursing and Midwifery Council's (ANMC) *Code of Ethics for Nurses in Australia* (2008) also states that nurses accept 'accountability for the standard of care they provide', including 'helping raise the standard of care, and taking action when they consider, on reasonable grounds, the standard of care is unacceptable. This includes a responsibility to question and report what they consider, on reasonable grounds, to be unethical treatment' (Value Statement 4).

It is important to clarify that for accountability to be fulfilled in nursing practice, clear standards of nursing care, and mechanisms for evaluating the accountability levels of nurses need to be developed (Johnstone 1998; Webster 1999). Standards for nursing practice give the nurse reference points for both self and peer evaluation of performance, and indicate a measure for accountability that can be used by nurse managers and administrators as well as nurse regulating authorities (nursing boards) concerned with monitoring and upholding professional standards of practice. This helps the nurse to understand what the profession and employers expect where accountability for practice is concerned. It also indicates a yardstick against which the practice of individual nurses can be measured, should they ever become the subject of a complaint or disciplinary proceeding (Johnstone 1998).

Obviously, accountability is a concept central to professional nursing practice, a concept from which important values are derived and principles formulated. Along with advocacy, accountability helps form a conceptual framework for the ethical dimensions of nursing practice.

Cooperation

Cooperation is a concept that, when applied in healthcare contexts encompasses the coordinated, collaborative, trust-based and productive interaction between members of the multi-professional health care team in the delivery of safe and high quality healthcare (Allwood, Traum & Jokinen 2000; Botes 2000). In practice, cooperation requires all 'co-operators' (the collection of individuals involved) to: (i) think about the other co-operators (cognitive consideration); (ii) have a joint purpose (i.e. each is aware of, has mutually contributed to and has agreed to work toward achieving the given purpose); (iii) take into account ethical considerations in regard to each other (i.e. will act ethically toward each other); and (iv) trust each other to act in accordance with all of the above three considerations (Allwood, Traum & Jokinen 2000; Uslaner 2002). Cooperation between a collection of individuals (even when unrelated) is widely considered to be beneficial, likely to maximise the interests of both individuals and the group, and critical to achieving long-term and sustainable goals (Allwood, Traum & Jokinen 2000; Theys & Kunsch 2004).

The responsibility of nurses to be 'cooperative' is clearly stated under Standard 4 of the ICN (2006) Code, notably: 'The nurse sustains a cooperative relationship with co-workers in nursing and other fields' (p. 3). The UK Nursing and Midwifery Council's (2002) *Code of Professional Conduct* likewise prescribes: 'As a registered nurse, midwife or specialist community public health nurse, you must cooperate with others in the team' (Standard 4). Other nursing codes also emphasise the responsibility of nurses to seek 'constructive and collaborative' approaches to team work, intra- and inter-professional communication, to resolving disagreement and conflict, and to contributing generally to 'the delivery of safe and quality care' (ANMC 2008, Value Statement 4) and to 'quality practice settings that are positive, healthy working environments' (CNA 2002, p. 18).

Cooperation fosters networks of mutual support and close working relationships (Lockhart-Wood 2000; Murphy 2000). The concept of cooperation supports such nursing actions as working with others toward shared goals, keeping promises, making mutual concerns a priority and sacrificing personal interests to the long-term maintenance of the professional relationship. All these actions express feelings traditionally valued by all human beings and support professional collaboration in designing and delivering safe and quality care to patients.

Nursing's historical documents and professional statements have often emphasised different aspects of professional cooperation. For example, Isabel Hampton Robb (1921, p. 139), an early nurse leader and scholar in the United States of America, linked cooperation to a special loyalty shared by members of the professional group:

'. . . she must remember that, for the time being, she is a member of a large family and its privacy and internal affairs should be as loyally guarded as those of her own home circle. The individuality of each member of the family should be respected; the shortcomings or mishaps of any nurse should never be made a topic of conversation outside, either to friends in the city or to doctors [. . .]. The principle of loyalty must be maintained, irrespective of personal feelings.'

The concept of cooperation has also been expressed as the power that enables professionals to work together. The writings of Florence Nightingale (Nutting & Dock 1907, pp. 277–278) emphasise this aspect of cooperation in the following passage:

'The health of the unit is the health of the community. Unless you have the health of the unit there is no community health. Competition, or each man [sic] for himself, and the devil against us all, may be necessary, we are told, but it is the enemy of health. Combination is the antidote – combined interests, recreation, combination to secure the best air, the best food, and all that makes life useful, healthy, and happy. There is no such thing as independence. As far as we are successful, our success lies in combination.'

Cooperation appears to form the basis of Nightingale's idea of human 'combination', maintaining and strengthening a community of nurses working toward a common goal. It does not mean that conflicts will not occur or that the good of patients should be sacrificed for the maintenance of the nurse's relationships with colleagues or with the employing institution. It does mean, however, that individual goals and interests might need to be compromised in order to achieve organisational and policy changes that will improve the safety and quality of patient care.

Cooperation is also an altruistic concept because it expresses the human bonds that grow from working together and spending time together (Fleming, Klein & Wilson 1999; Uslaner 2002). It can threaten patient care if one's relationships to members of the profession or co-workers become more important than the safety and quality of patient care. The appropriate role for cooperation, however, is the maintenance of working relationships and conditions that express obligations toward the patient and are mutually agreed upon. Cooperation can help unite nurses and other healthcare workers toward the shared goal of improved patient care (Quinn 1983). Along with advocacy and accountability, cooperation helps form a strong conceptual framework that enables nurses to meet the requirements of professional practice.

Caring

The ethical concept of caring has long been regarded as being foundational to the nurse–patient relationship and to the caring behaviours considered fundamental to the nursing role (Benner & Wrubel 1989; Leininger 1988; Watson 1985). The importance of caring in nursing is further underscored by its critical relationship to human health. As Leininger (1984) explains:

'The anthropologic record of the long survival of humans makes us pause to consider the role of care in the evolution of humankind. Different ecologic, cultural, social, and political contexts have influenced human health care and the survival of the human race. One can speculate that cultures could have destroyed themselves had not humanistic care acts helped to reduce intercultural stresses and conflicts and protect humans' (p. 5).

Nurse caring is specifically directed toward the protection of the health and welfare of patients. When caring is valued as important to the nursing role, it indicates a commitment toward certain patient outcomes, such as the protection of human dignity as well as the preservation of human health (Shiber & Larson 1991; Valentine 1991).

Others have defined caring as a moral obligation or duty among health professionals (Pellegrino 1985). Accordingly, one is obligated to promote the good of someone with whom one has a special relationship. The nurse–patient relationship is a 'special' relationship because it is created by the patient's need for nursing care. Nurses are obligated to show caring behaviours toward those in need of healthcare because doing so promotes patient good (Smerke 1990).

Caring can also be defined as a form of involvement with others that creates concern about how other individuals experience their world (Benner & Wrubel 1989). It requires 'sentiment and skills of connection and involvement, as well as caregiving, knowledge and skills' (Benner & Gordon 1996, p. 44). In one study of the experience of caring, four types of caring-as-involvement were identified: being there for the patient, respecting the patient, feeling with and for the patient, and closeness with the patient (Forrest 1989). All of these types of caring seem important to involvement with others and yield several distinct aspects of the phenomenon of caring. First, caring is a natural state of human existence, shared by every human being. It is the primary way that all humans relate to their world and to each other (Noddings 1984). As a natural sentiment of being human, caring is a feeling and an attitude that is universal for the whole human species. This is the type of caring that one commonly sees between a mother and child.

Second, caring is often a precondition of or an antecedent to caring *about* other entities. This aspect of caring is described by one author when she states that a conceptual idea about caring exists as a structural feature of human growth and development prior to the commencement of actual caring processes (Griffin 1983). One must have experience with caring before caring for something or someone else.

A third aspect of caring identifies it with moral or social ideals such as the human need to be protected from the elements or the need for love (Griffin 1983). Nursing practice is linked to these moral and social ideals because caring occurs within the context of healthcare which serves the needs of the community. Caring, therefore, is an ethical obligation and not simply a human behaviour (Smerke 1990). As an ethical obligation, its significance is always interpreted in terms of the special duties between individuals within a given context.

The degree to which caring behaviours can be implemented in nursing practice is influenced by several factors (Holden 1991). Nurse-related factors include such things as individual beliefs, educational experiences about caring, feeling good about nursing work and one's own experiences in caring for others or being cared for (Forrest 1989; Morse et al. 1991). The quality of nurse–patient communication is also a factor that influences nurse caring (Konishi & Davis 1999; Mendes, Trevizan, Nogueira & Sawada 1999). Patient-related factors include whether or not the patient is hard to care for or confirms the nurse's caring behaviours. Other factors that influence nurse caring include time to care, administrative support for caring behaviours, and the physical environment where care takes place (Forrest 1989; Johnstone 2001).

Some nurses have expressed concern about the extent to which nurses are expected to care for patients. For example, caring according to the ideal of care may result in nurses becoming physically and emotionally drained. According to some, too much caring may result in 'burnout' and nurse stress, may be unhealthy for both the nurse carer and the cared-for person, and may contribute to excessive nurse anxiety (Kuhse 1997). There is a potential personal cost to caring on the part of the nurse that has not been adequately understood or investigated. Yet, caring behaviours on the part of the nurse continue to be expected and valued by the profession and the public. Caring is universally considered fundamental to the nursing role, where human health is concerned, and its relevance to patient well-being continues to be analysed (Bradshaw 1999; Fry 1991; Sourial 1997).

Consensus on the concepts

Consensus on the moral concepts of nursing practice is increasing. Advocacy, for example, despite being a controversial concept, has long been supported in the nursing literature as a moral concept pertinent to the profession and practice of nursing (Gates 1994; Gaylord & Grace 1995; Grace 2001; MacDonald 2006; Sellin 1995; Snowball 1996). Linked with the virtues of courage and heroism, advocacy has been positioned as the means by which the nurse and the patient together determine the meaning that the experience of illness, suffering or dying may hold for that person (Gadow 1980, 1989). Advocacy has also been identified as the moral concept that defines how nurses view their responsibilities toward the patient (Chafey et al. 1998; Mallik 1997; Wheeler 2000).

The concept of moral accountability, championed by the North American nursing leader and scholar Lavinia Dock as early as 1900 (Johnstone 1999), has gained renewed attention as a critical moral foundation for nursing practice (Johnstone 1998; Hilbig & Manning 1999; Maas, Delaney & Huber 1999; Rowe 2000). The concept has been analysed in conjunction with the concept of responsibility (Johnstone 1998), and is now widely articulated in local and international codes of nursing ethics (e.g. ANA 2001; ANMC 2008; CNA 2002; ICN 2006; NMC 2004; SNB 2006).

The concept of cooperation has received broad support as a moral concept of nursing practice by its inclusion in local and international codes of nursing ethics (e.g. ANA 2001; ANMC 2008; CNA 2002; ICN 2006; NMC 2004). And although the notion of cooperation as a moral concept per se has not been widely discussed in the nursing literature, the importance and imperatives of creating effective teams and collaborative work relations in the workplace is being increasingly emphasised as being critical to the delivery of safe and quality care to patients (Higgins 1999; Johnstone 2007a, 2007b).

The concept of caring has long been claimed as a moral foundation for a nursing ethic that will protect and enhance the human dignity of patients receiving healthcare (Gadow 1985, 1999). Caring has also been described a moral art central to nursing and healthcare practices (Benner & Wrubel 1989; Watson 1985) as a way of knowing the patient (Benner & Gordon 1996), a moral virtue of nursing practice (Bradshaw 1999; Knowlden 1990) and as a moral ideal rooted in our notions of human dignity. All of these views position caring as a moral concept central to the nature of the nurse–patient relationship and the ethical practice of nursing.

Summary

The ethical concepts of advocacy, accountability, cooperation and caring have enjoyed a rich and distinctive history in nursing and will continue to have important implications for the future practice of nursing. Together, these concepts provide the foundation for ethical nursing actions and judgments, as well as professional standards and moral norms for nursing. They are important to public acceptance of nursing practice and are supported in professional codes of ethics and other written standards for nursing practice. However, administrative and professional support for these concepts is not universal. Hence, the degree to which these concepts can be upheld and strengthened in nursing practice during the twenty-first century will depend on several developments including: whether nurses obtain the legitimated authority they need to match their responsibilities as accountable and responsible health professionals; and the extent to which nurses recognise, accept, are educationally prepared and are willing to become involved politically to advocate and activate for the strategic policy and practice changes that are demonstrably needed to ensure that the universal right of all people to the highest attainable standard of health is realised.

References

Allwood, J., Traum, D. & Jokinen, K. (2000) Cooperation, dialogue and ethics. *Int J Human-Comput Stud* 53, 871–914.

American Nurses Association (2001) *Code of ethics for nurses with interpretive statements*. Washington, DC: ANA.

Australian Nursing and Midwifery Council (ANMC) (2008) *Code of ethics for nurses in Australia*. Canberra: ANMC.

Benner, P. & Gordon, S. (1996) Caring practice. In S. Gordon, S. Benner & N. Noddings (Eds) *Caregiving: Readings in knowledge, practice, ethics, & politics* (pp. 40–55). Philadelphia: University of Pennsylvania Press.

Benner, P. & Wrubel, J. (1989) *The primacy of caring*. Menlo Park, CA: Addison-Wesley.

Botes, A. (2000) An integrated approach to ethical decision-making in the health team. *J Adv Nurs* 32(5), 1076–1082.

Bradshaw, A. (1999) The virtue of nursing: The covenant of care. *J Med Ethics* 25, 477–481.

Canadian Nurses Association (CNA) (2002) *Code of ethics for registered nurses*. Ottawa, Ontario: Canadian Nurses Association.

Chafey, K., Rhea, M., Shannon, A.M. & Spencer, S. (1998) Characterizations of advocacy by practicing nurses. *J Prof Nurs* 14(1), 43–52.

Fleming, C. Klein, D. & Wilson, C. (1999) Forming collaborative relationships: Nurses and physicians unify their efforts with a single collaborative history and physical form. *Nurs Manage* 30(8), 38–39.

Forrest, D. (1989) The experience of caring. *J Adv Nurs* 14(10), 815–823.

Fry, S.T. (2004) Nursing ethics. In S.G. Post (Ed) *Encyclopedia of bioethics*, 3rd ed. (pp. 1898–1903). New York: Macmillan.

Fry, S.T. (1991) A theory of caring: Pitfalls and promises. In D.A. Gaut & M.M. Leininger (Eds) *Caring: The compassionate healer* (pp. 161–172). New York: National League for Nursing.

Fry-Revere, S. (1992) *The accountability of bioethics committees and consultants*. Frederick, MD: University Publishing Group, Inc.

Gadow, S. (1989) Clinical subjectivity: Advocacy for silent patients. *Nurs Clinics N Amer* 24(2), 535–541.

Gadow, S. (1980) Existential advocacy: Philosophical foundations of nursing. In S.F. Spicker & S. Gadow (Eds) *Nursing: Images and ideals* (pp. 79–101). New York: Springer.

Gadow, S. (1985) Nurse and patient: The caring relationship. In A. Bishop & J.R. Scudder, Jr. (Eds) *Caring, curing, coping: Nurse, physician, patient relationships* (pp. 31–43). Birmingham, AL: University of Alabama Press.

Gadow, S. (1999) Relational narrative: The postmodern turn in nursing ethics. *J Schol Inquiry* 13(1).

Gates, B. (1994) *Advocacy: A nurse's guide*. London: Scutari Press.

Gaylord, N. & Grace, P. (1995) Nursing advocacy: An ethic of practice. *Nurs Ethics* 2(1), 11–18.

Grace, P. (2001) Professional advocacy: widening the scope of accountability. *Nurs Philos* 2,151–162.

Griffin, A.P. (1983) A philosophical analysis of caring in nursing. *J Adv Nurs* 8, 289–295.

Henderson, V. (1977, rev. ed.) *Basic principles of nursing care.* Geneva: International Council of Nurses.

Higgins, L.W. (1999) Nurses' perceptions of collaborative nurse–physician transfer decision making as a predictor of patient outcomes in a medical intensive care unit. *J Adv Nurs* 29(6), 1434–1443.

Hilbig, J.I. & Manning, J. (1999) Accountability and responsibility underpins successful pain management. *J Perianesth Nurs* 14(6), 390–392.

Holden, R. (1991) An analysis of caring: Attributions, contributions and resolutions. *J Adv Nurs* 16, 893–898.

International Council of Nurses (ICN) (2006) *Code of ethics for nurses.* Geneva, Switzerland: ICN.

Jardin, K. Des. (2001) Political involvement in nursing – politics, ethics, and strategic action. *AORN J* 74(5), 614–628.

Johnstone, M.-J. (1998) *Determining and responding effectively to ethical professional misconduct in nursing: A report to the Nurses Board of Victoria.* Melbourne: RMIT University.

Johnstone, M.-J. (1999) *Bioethics: A nursing perspective,* 3rd ed. Sydney: Harcourt Saunders.

Johnstone, M.-J. (2001). Poor working conditions and the capacity of nurses to provide moral care. *Contemporary Nurse* 12(1), 7–15.

Johnstone, M.-J. (2004). *Bioethics: A nursing perspective,* 4th ed. Sydney: Elsevier Science.

Johnstone, M.-J. (2007a) Patient safety ethics and human error management in ED contexts, Part I: Development of the global patient safety movement. *Australasian Emergency Nurses Journal* 10(1), 13–20.

Johnstone, M.-J. (2007b) Patient safety ethics and human error management in ED contexts, Part II: Accountability and the challenge to change. *Australasian Emergency Nurses Journal* 10(2), 80–85.

Knowlden, V. (1990) The virtue of caring in nursing. In M.M. Leininger (Ed) *Ethical and moral dimensions of care* (pp. 89–94). Detroit: Wayne State University Press.

Konishi, E. & Davis, A.J. (1999) Japanese nurses' perceptions about disclosure of information at the patients' end of life. *Nurs & Hlth Serv* 1, 179–187.

Kuhse, K. (1997) *Caring: Nursing, women, and ethics.* Oxford/Cambridge, Mass: Blackwell Pub.

Leininger, M.M. (1984) Care: The essence of nursing and health. In *Care: The essence of nursing and health,* pp. 3–15. Detroit: Wayne State University Press.

Leininger, M.M. (Ed) (1988) *Care: The essence of nursing and health,* pp. 3–15. Detroit: Wayne State University Press.

Lockhart-Wood, K. (2000) Specialist nursing: Collaboration between nurses and doctors in clinical practice. *Br J Nurs* 9(5), 276–280.

Maas, M.L., Delaney, D. & Huber, D. (1999) Nursing outcomes accountability: Contextual variables and assessment of the outcome effects of nursing interventions. *Outcomes Manage Nurs Pract* 3(1), 4–6.

MacDonald, H. (2006) Relational ethics and advocacy in nursing: Literature review. *J Adv Nurs* 57(2), 119–126.

McMurray, A. (1991) Advocacy for community self-empowerment. *Int. Nurs Rev* 38(1), 19–21.

Mallik, M. (1997) Advocacy in nursing: Perceptions of practising nurses. *J Clin Nurs* 6, 303–313.

Mendes, I.A., Trevizan, M.A., Nogueira, M.S. & Sawada, N.O. (1999) Humanizing nurse-patient communication: A challenge and commitment. *Med Law* 18, 639–644.

Morrison, P. (1989) Nursing and caring: A personal construct theory study of some nurses' self-perceptions. *J Adv Nurs* 14(5), 421–426.

Morse, J. Bottorff, J. Neander, W. & Solberg, S. (1991) Comparative analysis of concep-
tualisations and theories of caring. *Image: J Nurs Sch* 23(2), 119–126.

Murphy, F.A. (2000) Collaborating with practitioners in teaching and research: A model
for developing the role of the nurse lecturer in practice areas. *J Adv Nurs* 31(3), 704–714.

Noddings, N. (1984) *Caring: A feminine approach to ethics and moral education.*
Berkeley, CA: University of California Press.

Nursing Council of Hong Kong (1999) *Code of Professional Conduct and Code of Ethics
for Nurses in Hong Kong.* Hong Kong: Nursing Council of Hong Kong.

Nursing and Midwifery Council (NMC) (2004) *Code of professional conduct.* London:
Nursing and Midwifery Council (UK).

Nutting, M.A. & Dock, L.L. (1907) *A history of nursing*, vol. 2. New York: G.P.
Putnam's Sons.

Otto, D.A. (1999) Regulatory statutes and issues: Clinical accountability in perioper-
ative settings. *AORN J* 70(2), 241–244, 246–247, 249–252.

Page, A. (Ed) (2004) *Keeping patients safe: Transforming the work environments of nurses.*
Washington, DC: The National Academies Press.

Pellegrino, E. (1985) The caring ethic: The relation of physician to patient. In A.H. Bishop
& J.R. Scudder (Eds) *Caring, curing, coping: Nurse, physician, patient relationships*
(pp. 8–30). Birmingham, AL: University of Alabama Press.

Quinn, S. (Ed) (1983) *Cooperation and conflict: Caring for the carers.* Geneva:
International Council of Nurses.

Robb, I.H. (1921) *Nursing ethics: For hospital and private use.* Cleveland, OH: E.C. Koeckert.

Rowe, J.A. (2000) Accountability: A fundamental component of nursing practice.
B J Nurs 9(9), 549–552.

Sellin, S.C. (1995) Out on a limb: A qualitative study of patient advocacy in institutional
nursing. *Nurs Ethics* 2(1), 19–29.

Shiber, S. & Larson, E. (1991) Evaluating the quality of caring: Structure, process and
outcome. *Holistic Nurs Prac* 5(3), 57–66.

Singapore Nursing Board (2006) *Code of ethics and professional conduct.* Singapore:
Singapore Nursing Board.

Smerke, J. (1990) Ethical components of caring. *Crit Care Nurs Clin N Amer* 2(3), 509–513.

Snowball, J. (1996) Asking nurses about advocating for patients: Reactive and proactive
accounts. *J Adv Nurs* 24, 67–75.

Sourial, S. (1997) An analysis of caring. *J Adv Nurs* 26, 1189–1192.

Theys, M. & Kunsch, P. (2004) The importance of co-operation for ethical decision-
making with OR. *European Journal of Operational Research* 153, 485–488.

Uslaner, E. (2002) *The moral foundations of trust.* Cambridge, UK: Cambridge
University Press.

Valentine, K. (1991) Comprehensive assessment of caring and its relationship to outcome
measures. *J Nurs Qual Ass* 5(2), 59–68.

Watson, J. (1985) *Nursing: the philosophy and science of caring.* Boulder, CO:
Associated University Press.

Webster, J. (1999) Practitioner/centered research: An evaluation of the implementation
of the bedside hand-over. *J Adv Nurs* 30(6), 1375–1382.

Wheeler, P. (2000) Is advocacy at the heart of professional practice? *Nurs Stan* 14(36),
39–41.

Chapter 4
Standards of ethical conduct in nursing

Standards of ethical conduct in nursing have been strongly influenced by the various historical, social and cultural contexts in which they – and the profession of nursing itself – have been developed (Heikkinen et al. 2006; Johnstone 1994, 2004). Historically, the professional conduct and practice of nursing was primarily guided by the principles and standards of etiquette (style and decorum), not ethics, and by unwritten conventions and 'customs' governing the behaviour of 'good woman' in public domains (Johnstone 1993, 1999). As the profession of nursing developed, however, and its moral goals to promote health, prevent illness, restore health and alleviate suffering were made more explicit, the standards of ethical conduct in nursing likewise developed. Whereas rules of etiquette (both written and unwritten) once stood as the ultimate standards of professional nursing conduct, statements of principled moral action were gradually set forth in formal codes of nursing ethics and ultimately surpassed etiquette as the primary prescription for and measure of ethical conduct in nursing.

Early standards for nurses' ethical behaviours

Ethical behaviour of the nurse was associated very early with the image of the nurse as a 'good woman' in service to others. Despite the significant nurse education reforms that were spearheaded by Florence Nightingale in England and others elsewhere, it was generally assumed that in order to be a 'good nurse' all one had to be was a 'good woman'. A good nurse, in this instance, was someone who had responded to a vocational calling to be a nurse and who was committed to the high ideal of doing what was 'right'. Being of the highest class of character, the 'good nurse' (good woman) was always chaste, sober, honest, truthful, trustworthy, punctual, modest, quiet and cheerful (Nutting & Dock 1907; see also Johnstone 1993). Such a nurse, disciplined by her moral training, could be relied upon to do her duty in serving others, including obediently following the orders of her superiors.

This view of the nurse as a good woman is echoed in several early 'nursing ethics' texts, such as Robb's *Nursing Ethics* (1921). In addition to being physically and morally strong, the nurse, according to Robb, must be a dignified, cultured, courteous, well-educated and reserved woman of good breeding. Robb considered the nurse's work a service to others that was performed in the spirit of religious duty. Thus through the writings of medical men and various nurse leaders, published either as texts or as articles in nursing periodicals, moral virtue, moral duty and service to others became established as the foundation on which standards for nurses' ethical behaviour would be built.

During the early twentieth century, being ethical in nursing practice meant primarily following nursing etiquette and established customs or conventions of socially acceptable behaviour (Johnstone 1993). Nursing etiquette included forms of polite behaviour such as neatness, punctuality, courtesy and quiet attendance on the physician. It also included an attitude of deference to authority figures, especially the nursing supervisor and the physician. The performance of duty included strict adherence to the rules of the institution and an attitude of self-sacrifice. The nurse demonstrated her moral duty by being loyal to the physician, her training school and the institution (Fry 2004). Unquestioning obedience and minding one's own affairs were additional means by which the nurse demonstrated the acceptance of her moral duties (Robb 1921).

Although there was a strong emphasis on etiquette in early nursing texts, some authors recognised that there was also an overlap between etiquette and ethics as standards of ethical behaviour. For example, nursing ethics is described by Aikens (1931) as the ideals, customs and habits associated with the general characteristics of a nurse. Gladwin (1930) viewed nursing ethics as doing one's duty with skill and moral perfection. Robb (1921) defined nursing ethics as the rules of conduct followed by the nurse while attending to the sick. Textbooks published as late as the 1950s likewise admonished the nurse to conduct her professional relationships with loyalty, prudence, desirable personality and respectful conduct (Morison 1957). However, some important distinctions between etiquette and ethics were understood. For example, whereas etiquette was accepted as being necessary in order to ensure professional harmony in patient care, ethics was deemed to be critical for ensuring moral excellence, technical competence and moral responsibility and accountability in nursing practice (Dock 1900). On this point one early US nurse leader, Lavinia Dock, went even further and famously argued that not only must nurses be ethical but that, in order to be ethical and to be able to fulfil their moral responsibilities as professional women, nurses needed *to be free* – to have 'the same amount of independence as any other moral being' (Dock 1900, pp. 41 & 49). Anything less, she contended, would be to risk the moral cowardice of subordination and the slavishness of blind obedience (Dock 1900, pp. 41 & 49).

Over time, the nurse's role in patient care slowly shifted from being the obedient helper of the physician to being an independent practitioner who was and could be held independently accountable for what had been done (or not done) in providing patient care. This shift in roles was accompanied by a shift in viewpoints about acceptable ethical standards of conduct for nurses. No longer would the nurse's moral responsibilities be couched solely in terms of obedience to authority and loyalty to the physician, hospital and co-workers. Changing values in society began to affect how nurses conceptualised their responsibilities toward patients, co-workers and their employing institutions (Fry 2004; Johnstone 1993, 1994). Rather than just carrying out ethical decisions made by others, the nurse began to claim authority for independent nursing decisions in patient care, including ethical decisions.

Development of nursing codes of ethics

A code can be defined as 'a conventionalized set of rules or expectations devised for a select purpose' (Johnstone 2004, p. 19). During the first part of the twentieth century, the need for a code of ethics for nursing practice was discussed by professional nursing organisations throughout the world (Freitas 1990). However, it was not until the middle of the century that codes of ethics for nurses would be accepted by various nursing organisations. In some cases, it was not until the 1990s that codes of ethics for nurses were developed, disseminated, implemented and promoted in the contexts in which they had been formulated (Heikkinen et al. 2006; Verpeet et al. 2005, 2006).

The International Council of Nurses (ICN) began working toward the development of a code of ethics for all nurses in the world at the 1923 ICN Congress held in Montreal, Canada (Quinn 1989). Work on the development of a code of ethics was interrupted by World War II, but the ICN's Ethics of Nursing Committee nonetheless produced a draft of an International Code of Nursing Ethics at the 1953 ICN Congress held in Sao Paulo, Brazil. The ICN Code for Nurses was accepted at the 1953 Congress and immediately translated into other languages besides English, as well as being printed in a small size pocket form for distribution to member nurses' associations (Quinn 1989). The Code was revised in 1965 and 1973, and a publication on the use of the Code in nursing practice was produced by the ICN in 1977. The 1973 version was reconfirmed by the ICN Professional Services Committee in 1989. In 2000, the Code was revised and retitled as The Code of Ethics for Nurses. The Code was again reviewed, revised and reaffirmed in 2005 (ICN 2006).

A significant number of national nurses' associations throughout the world (e.g. Australia, Canada, Denmark, Finland, France, Germany, Greece, Hong King, Italy, the Netherlands, New Zealand, Poland, Romania, Singapore, South Africa, Switzerland, Spain, the UK, the USA, to name some) have developed a code of ethics for their members or are in the process of developing one (Biton & Tabak 2003; Heikkinen et al. 2006; Johnstone 2004; Verpeet et al. 2005, 2006). While the majority of national nurses' associations use the ICN *Code of Ethics for Nurses* (2006), other associations have developed their own codes of ethics. Many of these codes, although developed independently, are closely aligned with the ICN Code.

Purpose of a code of ethics

According to Johnstone (1998), codes of ethics serve several purposes. One purpose is to foster and maintain ethical standards of professional conduct. A code may do this by cultivating moral character and encouraging a person to engage in self-conscious moral reflection. A code may also prescribe conduct that is not amenable to legislation, conduct such as voluntarily engaging in ethical behaviour and caring for, and about, patients. A second function of a code is to regulate ethical professional conduct and to provide a tool for evaluating the ethical competence of nurses. It sets the parameters of acceptable ethical practice and demonstrates to the public what is required of nurses. It also proclaims the standards of ethical practice that all nurses are required to meet and provides nurses with a 'professional compass' (Biton & Tabak 2003; Heikkinen et al. 2006) for guiding 'right' decision making in their work.

Spicer (1995) points out that moral guidelines in a code of ethics generally involve three elements: values, duties and virtues. Values denote the primary good or objective espoused by the profession. In nursing, this might be patient well-being. Duties are usually broad in nature and identify behaviours that people are 'bound' to perform for moral reasons, such as respect human dignity, preserve people's capacity for self-determination, maintain confidentiality, and so forth. Virtues in a code can include character traits that are desired in the members of the professional group. In nursing, this might be honesty, compassion, truthfulness and personal integrity.

The functions and moral guidelines of a code outlined above are relevant to nursing codes of ethics. Many early codes of ethics for nursing did, in fact, emphasise the personal conduct of the nurse, and projected the ethical image of the professional nurse to the public at large. Later codes of ethics emphasised the responsibility of the nurse to the patient and the maintenance of nursing practice standards. Values, duties and the virtues of nurses can be seen in nursing codes' requirements to keep patient information confidential, be accountable for nursing actions and to respect the dignity and rights of all people, and to take action in instances where the rights of people are being violated or are at risk of being violated to the detriment of their health and well-being.

Common themes in nursing codes of ethics

Common themes in contemporary nursing codes of ethics include the nurse's relations with co-workers; the nurse's responsibility to report the incompetence of other healthcare workers; the nurse's accountability in delegating functions to others; the obligation to respect the life and dignity of the patient; the nurse's responsibility for maintenance of patient confidentiality. Additionally, non-discrimination against persons based on cultural background, nationality, creed, race, colour, religion, socioeconomic status, gender, sexual orientation or political beliefs, and the need to safeguard the patient from harm, are common (Figure 4.1)

Professional issues
- practice competence and relations with co-workers
- conditions of employment
- purpose of nursing profession and personal conduct
- incompetence of other healthcare workers
- responsibility of the nurse to develop knowledge and standards for the profession
- role and accountability of the nurse when delegating functions to others

Patient issues
- respect life and dignity of the patient
- uphold patient confidentiality
- nondiscrimination against persons because of cultural background, nationality, creed, race, colour, religion, socioeconomic status, gender, sexual orientation or political beliefs
- safety of the patient; safeguarding from harm

Societal issues
- addressing and improving the health and social needs of the community
- ethical guidelines for research
- nurse's relation to the state and obeying laws of country
- euthanasia and assisted suicide

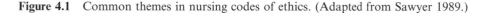

Figure 4.1   Common themes in nursing codes of ethics. (Adapted from Sawyer 1989.)

(Sawyer 1989). Several professional codes mention the patient advocacy role of the nurse, the obligation to respect the autonomy of patients, the nurse's role in promoting patient access to healthcare, the nurse's accountability to the patient and respect for patients' values. Many codes of ethics address the nurse's relation to the state and the obligation to obey the laws of the country as well as the nurse's role in euthanasia and natural or human-made disasters. A few codes of ethics explicitly state that nurses should not be involved in torture and abortion (Sawyer 1989). More recently, the issues of clinical risk management and a systems approach to patient safety and human error management in healthcare, being responsive to cultural and linguistic diversity in healthcare, respecting indigenous peoples and promoting the collective responsibility of communities to promote reconciliation between Aboriginal and 'newcomer' populations, whistle-blowing, bullying in the workplace, the interrelationship between health and human rights, have all been made more explicit as areas in which nurses have particular ethical responsibilities (see, for example, the ANMC revised code).

The most common areas of agreement in nursing codes of ethics are nursing responsibility for practice competence, the need for good relations with co-workers, respect for the life and dignity of the patient, protection of patient confidentiality and the nurse's moral position of non-discrimination where patients are concerned (Sawyer 1989). These areas of agreement are often found in other professional codes of ethics.

In the ICN *Code of Ethics for Nurses* (2006), important aspects of nursing practice are grouped under four major headings:

(1)   nurses and people (those who require nursing care)
(2)   nurses and practice (personal responsibility and accountability)

(3) nurses and the profession (implementing standards of nursing practice and working conditions)
(4) nurses and co-workers (sustaining cooperative relationships)

The ethical responsibilities of the nurse are clearly stated: to promote health, to prevent illness, to restore health and to alleviate suffering. The ICN interprets the *Code of Ethics for Nurses* to be 'a guide for action based on social values and needs' (ICN 2006, p. 4). It serves as a practical aid in choosing priorities of action and the scope of such action in specific situations involving ethical questions or unethical behaviour on the part of co-workers and/or institutions. Applications of the *Code of Ethics for Nurses* by practitioners and managers, educators and researchers, and national nurses' associations are illustrated in publications of the *Code of Ethics for Nurses*. The ICN encourages nurses to help with the dissemination of the *Code of Ethics for Nurses* to schools of nursing, practising nurses, the nursing press, the media, the public, consumers, policy makers and employers of nurses.

Like all professional codes of ethics, nursing codes provide important ethical standards that nurses can refer to for both self-evaluation and peer review of professional ethical practice and when faced with ethical questions during the course of their work. Codes can also help 'with the cultivation of moral character' (Johnstone 2004, p. 21). This they can do by 'increasing the probability that people will behave in some ways rather than others' – specifically that they will behave in the 'right way' and for the 'right reasons' (Lichtenberg 1996, p. 15). Thus, although codes may have limited legal authority (Johnstone 1994, 2004) they can nonetheless provide nurses with a reason to think and act ethically, notably by reminding them 'of the moral point of the sorts of activities they are involved in' as members of the nursing profession (Coady 1996, p. 286; Johnstone 2004, p. 21).

Application and enforcement of nursing codes of ethics

Like all professional codes of ethics, nursing codes may prove difficult to apply to and in patient care situations (Biton & Tabak 2003; Heikkinen et al. 2006; Johnstone 1994, 2004). Since their statements represent moral values and ideals rather than specific behaviours that should be carried out by the nurse, some professional nursing organisations have developed lengthy interpretations of nursing codes of ethics (ANA 2001; CNA 2002) or produced textbooks of case applications of a code (this text, commissioned by the ICN, being a case in point).

Historically, codes of professional ethics have been difficult to enforce. It has even been argued that one's personal moral code provides a stronger basis for ethical judgments and actions made in the professional role than any code of ethics can ever hope to provide (Fry & Veatch 2006). Nurses may, however, experience conflict in trying to balance their personal values with the professional values and duties required by a code and, moreover, may discover that their personal and 'ordinary moral apparatus' for dealing with ethical issues in the workplace is not always adequate on account of the complexity of the ethical issues often encountered in professional contexts (Osei-Boateng 1998; Johnstone 1994, 1998, 2004).

The legitimated authority of professional nursing codes is, however, beginning to change as is evident by their increasing use as a 'tool for peer review' by managers and disciplinary boards in instances where a nurse's conduct is called into question. Moreover, there is an emerging consensus that it would be desirable for the ethical behaviours mandated by a code to be disseminated more widely than has traditionally been done, and for them even to be incorporated into the policies and guidelines of employer organisations so that their application to and in nursing practice can be facilitated (Biton & Tabak 2003; Johnstone 2001; Verpeet et al. 2005, 2006).

A professional code of ethics has long been recognised as an important hallmark of a profession (Fry & Veatch 2006; Johnstone 2004). Accordingly, the development, dissemination, implementation, and enforcement of professional codes of ethics in nursing have been given considerable attention and thought throughout the world. As the complexities of ethical nursing practice become more evident, and the need to have reliable processes in place to help navigate and negotiate morally wise solutions to the issues encountered in everyday practice, it is likely that discussion and debate about the role and content of codes of nursing ethics will continue.

Summary

Standards of ethical professional conduct in nursing have evolved, as has the profession and discipline of nursing, throughout the past century. At one time, a nurse's adherence to ethical standards meant obedience to the physician and loyalty to the hospital; now, however, it means following ethical principles and standards of conduct set forth in professional codes of ethics. The International Council of Nurses' *Code of Ethics for Nurses* (2006) has been the model for professional codes of ethics in countries throughout the world. This code supports ethical standards for nursing practice such as nursing responsibilities: to people (individuals, families, communities) requiring nursing care; to uphold the standards of responsible and accountable nursing practice; to respect the life and dignity of people; and to ensure that people are not discriminated against or treated in a way that violates their rights to and in healthcare.

References

Aikens, C.S. (1931) *Studies in ethics for nurses.* Philadelphia: W.B. Saunders.
American Nurses Association (ANA) (2001) *Code of ethics for nurses with interpretative statements.* Washington, DC: ANA.

Australian Nursing and Midwifery Council (2007) *Code of ethics for nurses in Australia.* Canberra: Australian Nursing and Midwifery Council.

Biton, V. & Tabak, N. (2003) The relationship between the application of the nursing ethical code and nurses' work satisfaction. *International Journal of Nursing Practice* 9, 140–157.

Canadian Nurses' Association (CNA) (2002) *Code of ethics for registered nurses.* Ottawa, Ontario: CNA.

Coady, C. (1996) On regulating ethics. In M. Coady and S. Bloch (Eds) *Codes of ethics and the professions* (pp. 269–287). Melbourne: Melbourne University Press.

Dock, L.L. (1900) Ethics – or a code of ethics? In L.L. Dock *Short papers on nursing subjects.* New York: M. Louise Longeway.

Freitas, L. (1990) Historical roots and future perspectives related to nursing ethics. *J Prof Nurs* 6(4), 197–205.

Fry, S.T. (2004) Nursing ethics. In S.G. Post (Ed) *Encyclopedia of bioethics*, 3rd ed (pp. 1898–1903). New York: Macmillan.

Fry, S.T. & Veatch, R.M. (2006) *Case studies in nursing ethics*, 3rd ed. Boston: Jones and Bartlett.

Gladwin, M.E. (1930) *Ethics: Talks to nurses.* Philadelphia: W.B. Saunders.

Heikkinen, A., Lemonidou, C., Petsios, K., Sala, R., Barazzetti, G., Radealli, S. & Leino-Kilpi, H. (2006) Ethical codes in nursing practice: the viewpoint of Finnish, Greek and Italian nurses. *J Adv Nurs* 55(3), 310–319.

International Council of Nurses (ICN) (2006) *Code of ethics for nurses.* Geneva, Switzerland: ICN.

Johnstone, M.-J. (1993) The development of nursing ethics in Australia: A historical overview. *Proceedings of the First National Nursing History Conference: Australian nursing: The story* (pp. 33–51). Canberra: Royal College of Nursing, Australia.

Johnstone, M.-J. (1994) *Nursing and the injustices of the law.* Sydney: WB Saunders/Baillière Tindall.

Johnstone, M.-J. (1998) *Determining and responding effectively to ethical professional misconduct in nursing: A report to the Nurses Board of Victoria.* Melbourne: RMIT University.

Johnstone, M.-J. (1999) Be good women but do not bother with a code of ethics. *Bioethics: A nursing perspective*, 3rd ed (ch. 2). Sydney: Harcourt Saunders.

Johnstone, M.-J. (2001) Poor working conditions and the capacity of nurses to provide moral care. *Contemporary Nurse* 12(1), 7–15.

Johnstone, M.-J. (2004) *Bioethics: A nursing perspective*, 4th ed. Sydney: Churchill Livingstone/Elsevier.

Lichtenberg, J. (1996) What are codes of ethics for? In M. Coady and S. Bloch (Eds) *Codes of ethics and the professions* (pp. 13–27). Melbourne: Melbourne University Press.

Morison, L.J. (1957) *Steppingstones to professional nursing.* St. Louis, MO: C.V. Mosby.

Nutting, M.A. & Dock, L.L. (1907) *A history of nursing*, vol. 2. New York: G.P. Putnam's Sons.

Osei-Boateng, M. (1998) Evolution and problems of nursing ethics. *W Afr J Nurs* 9(1), 15–20.

Quinn, D.S. (1989) *ICN: Past and present.* Middlesex, England: Scutari Press.

Robb, I.H. (1921) *Nursing ethics: For hospital and private use.* Cleveland, OH: E.C. Koeckert.

Sawyer, L.M. (1989) Nursing code of ethics: An international comparison. *Intl Nurs Rev* 36(5), 145–148.

Spicer, C.A. (1995) Nature and role of codes and other ethics directives. In W.T. Reich (Ed) *Encyclopedia of Bioethics*, 2nd ed (pp. 33597–33704). New York: Macmillan.

Verpeet, E., de Casterlé, B., Van der Arend, A. & Gastmans, C. (2005) Nurses' views on ethical codes: a focus group study. *J Adv Nurs* 51(2), 188–195.

Verpeet, E., de Casterlé, B., Lemiengre, J. & Gastmans, C. (2006) Belgian nurses' views on codes of ethics: development, dissemination, implementation. *Nurs Ethics* 13(5), 531–545.

Chapter 5
Ethical analysis and decision making in nursing practice

The ability to make ethical decisions is essential to moral excellence in professional nursing practice (Fry 2004). To foster development of this ability, the majority of nursing education programmes throughout the world offer some course content in ethics (see Appendix 1 for approaches to teaching ethics). Nursing education also encourages students to develop moral vision and moral imagination (Scott 1997), as well as moral intuition (Easen & Wilcockson 1996), critical thinking skills (Maynard 1996) and political savvy (Johnstone 2004).

One goal of ethics teaching is to produce a morally informed, knowledgeable, sensitive and accountable nurse who has the ability to make ethical decisions in practice (Fry 2004; Oddi, Cassidy & Fisher 1995). Another goal is to prepare future practitioners of nursing who are able to identify and respond effectively to ethical issues in nursing and healthcare contexts (Johnstone 1998, 2004). To achieve these goals, students must learn to integrate their personal values and beliefs with knowledge of ethical concepts, approaches to ethics and standards for ethical behaviour. This integration will then become part of the nurse's framework for making ethical decisions and implementing them in patient care (Figure 5.1).

Models for ethical analysis and decision making

Ethicists recognise that there are many components and variables in decision making, and that no single decision-making method is appropriate or useful for everyone. However, ethical decision making can be enhanced by an orderly process that considers the methods of ethics (as discussed in Chapter 2), and the context within which ethical questions arise in patient care. Different models of ethical decision making represent the various systematic processes or approaches

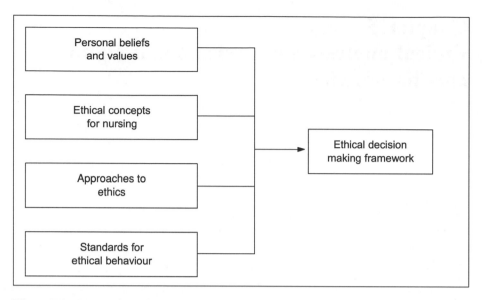

Figure 5.1   Integration of essential content for ethical decision making.

that a nurse might take in making an ethical decision related to the health and nursing care of an individual or a population group. These models are useful in helping the decision maker examine:

(1)   the values involved and the interests at stake
(2)   the context within which the decision will be made
(3)   the kinds of strategies that will need to be employed to achieve a resolution to the problems identified
(4)   the nature of the nurse's responsibilities in the situation.

They do not provide a foolproof formula for arriving at the 'right' decision. There is no perfect recipe for ethical decision making in nursing practice. Each nurse brings his or her own knowledge of ethics and values, life experiences, cognitive abilities, moral sensitivity, reasoning abilities and personal moral motivations to the process of making an ethical decision and acting on it.

Ethical decision making is a systematic process that is often formally taught in nursing education. Course content in ethics usually includes exposure to ethical decision making models and their application in analysing and resolving ethical issues in hypothetical patient care situations. Used in conjunction with a knowledge of the discipline of ethics, models thus promote development of the abilities required for ethical nursing practice.

A number of ethical decision making models for use in nursing have been proposed. All provide an orderly approach to analysing both the 'factual' and value dimensions involved in ethical conflicts and offer a systematic approach to implementing ethical decisions in patient care. Some are skeletal guidelines while others offer a more detailed approach to ethical decision making.

1. Recognise moral dimensions of the task or problem

2. Enumerate the guiding and evaluative principles

3. Specify the stakeholders and their guiding principles

4. Plot various action alternatives

5. Evaluate alternatives in light of principles and stakeholders

6. Consult and involve stakeholders as appropriate

7. Tell stakeholders the reasons for the decision

Figure 5.2   RESPECT model for ethical analyses and decision making. (Yeo & Moorhouse 1996, p. 381; used with permission.)

A few models closely resemble the problem-solving or nursing process approach taught in some schools of nursing (Davis, Aroskar, Liaschenko & Drought 1997; Johnstone 2004). One model combines the problem-solving process in nursing with a theological perspective (Shelly 2000). Another model combines a problem-solving approach with a business perspective (Yeo & Moorhouse 1996). Called the RESPECT model, it is oriented to the 'stakeholder' or the person who will be most affected by a decision and is, therefore, entitled to have his or her interests and values considered and respected in the decision-making process (Figure 5.2).

Other models help the nurse explore and analyse the context within which the value conflict has arisen and the views of the key parties to the decision without presupposing that traditional ethical principles will automatically 'apply' to the situation. Johnstone's (2004) moral decision making model, for example, includes a five-step process that guides:

(1) a critically reflective assessment of the situation
(2) the identification and 'diagnosis' of moral problems
(3) planning an appropriate course of action to address the problem(s) identified
(4) implementing the plan of action
(5) evaluating the moral outcomes of the action(s) taken can be used to clarify the nature of a problem and then solve it (Figure 5.3)

Nurses should not feel that one, and only one, model works best in all situations. It is likely that differences in patient care situations will require different approaches to ethical problems depending on the values of the decision maker, the nurse and other parties involved.

The majority of ethical problems faced by the nurse are important but not necessarily complex. They are situations involving conflicts of values in fairly routine patient care situations. They become interesting and morally complex, however, when the values involved arise from strongly held cultural, religious and moral beliefs. Therefore, a values-centred model of ethical decision making is offered here that can be used in conjunction with other models or used alone, depending on the situation.

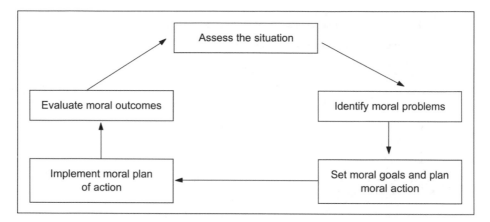

Figure 5.3   Johnstone's moral decision making model (2004).

A model for ethical analysis and decision making in nursing practice

The following model (Figure 5.4) uses four questions to help the nurse:

1. What is the story behind the value conflicts?
2. What is the significance of the values involved?
3. What is the significance of this conflict to the parties involved?
4. What should be done?

Figure 5.4   Model for ethical analysis and decision making.

1.   What is the story behind the value conflicts?

By asking this question, the nurse begins to discover how the problem is defined by the parties experiencing the problem. The story needs to be told by each of the parties involved in terms of factual information (who did what), in terms of the values of the parties involved (why the situation is seen as an ethical problem) and the conflicts of values perceived by the parties involved (Mattison 2000). It is important to allow the telling of the story in all its dimensions and through the eyes of all parties involved – the patient, the family members or other caregivers, the nurse, the attending medical practitioner(s), other allied healthcare workers, administrative officials, etc. When the full story of the problem is known, the context within which the problem arose will be made explicit and the various interpretations of the problem and the values of the parties involved will become clear. In this way the value conflicts will be clarified. Ethical problems always involve conflicts of moral values with other values (moral and nonmoral).

2. What is the significance of the values involved?

In exploring the meaning of the values held by the parties involved, one gains insight into the moral and nonmoral nature of the values and their potential cultural, religious, personal, professional and even political origins (Raines 2000). Additional questions that might need to be asked include: What does it mean to 'care' for this patient and what are my nursing responsibilities to this patient? Are there any legal questions that might need to be explored by a legal representative? How do I, as a professional nurse, maintain my ethical integrity in this situation?

Exploring the significance of the values held by individuals in any situation is always very important (Mariano 2001). Ethical problems cannot be adequately resolved unless the value dimensions of the problem are known, respected and considered in the decision-making process. This does not mean that all values will always be protected. In fact, in most conflicts the nurse plays a crucial role in assisting parties involved to examine their values and the values of others so that the parties can begin to negotiate. In other words, the parties to the conflict will need to decide which values are most important to preserve and protect, and which values might be of lesser importance. The goal of the professional nurse is to help the parties involved to respect each other's values and to help individuals prioritise their values and preserve the most important ones in the process of decision making. This can only be done when the significance of all values involved is known.

3. What is the significance of this conflict to the parties involved?

In answering this question, the nurse learns how the parties involved relate their values to the present situation. Values are never static. They are dynamic in that they change over time and in relation to significant human events and relationships. Situations of value conflicts likewise do not occur in a vacuum. They have a history and a necessary social, economic and political content that make them significant or nonsignificant to the parties involved. The conflicts of values might lead to a decision that affects the quality of a person's life, how long she or he might live, the amount of guilt that other parties to the conflict might experience, the emotional and psychological stress that individuals might experience following the resolution of the conflict and the nurse's professional demeanour and standing.

The acknowledgement of conflicts of values might also lead to the formation of policy that helps to resolve or prevent such value conflicts from occurring in the future. The nature of the value conflicts might have great significance for health professionals who often must deal repeatedly with conflicts of values in the work environment (Baggs et al. 1997; Berggren, Barbosa da Silva & Severinsson 2005). Exploring the significance of the value conflicts to the parties involved can help nurses and other health professionals to formulate policy and policy changes before more complex ethical situations arise in patient care.

4.   What should be done?

By asking this question, the nurse explores all of the ways in which the value conflicts might be resolved. Sometimes consensus might be reached relatively quickly on what constitutes the 'right thing to do'; other times, there may be no 'ethically correct' solution to the problem at hand. In most cases, ethical decisions are made based on the amount of relevant information available at that time, the significance (moral weight) of the value dimensions and the 'best' judgment of the decision maker(s) or the collective ethical stance of the group. Knowing a variety of possible ways in which the conflicts might be resolved gives the involved parties options to explore. These options should be explored in light of:

(1)   the values held by the various parties
(2)   outcomes that may occur
(3)   the moral rightness or wrongness of the various options according to agreed moral standards

Some options might be ethically permissible, i.e. do not conflict with the professional code of ethics, but may not support the values of the key decision maker(s), other parties to the situation or the community group consensus. Some options might not be ethically permissible although they might support important values. On the other hand, some options might be ethically permissible for the patient, family members or caregivers, or community group (i.e. consistent with their personal, cultural, and religious and personal values) but not be permissible for attending health professionals.

At some point, the key decision maker(s) must choose a course of action based on their considered best judgments about what ought to be done. This decision is often very individual but is morally responsive in that it stems from a careful consideration of the context of the value conflicts, the values of all parties involved, the ethical relevance of these values, and the moral meaning of the situation to individuals involved. It is also a reasoned decision, based on a careful process of ethical reflection and supported by ethical principles (Rhodes 2000).

Following the implementation of the choice or decision made, some assessment should be made about the outcome of the situation and the process that led to the decision. The nurse should always consider whether the process could have been improved and what implications, if any, the conflicts of values have for future patient care situations (Otto & Kennedy-Schwarz 2000). Engaging in reflection enables one to learn from the ethical experience and to improve future practice (Johns 1999; Woods 1999).

Nurses who deliver specialised nursing care (midwifery, critical or trauma care, maternal/newborn care, care to cancer patients, elderly persons or those who are dying, etc.) often see the same or similar value conflicts recurring time after time. If these conflicts are related to the nature of the medical problem, the cultural or religious belief systems of the patients or the personal or professional values of the healthcare workers, the way in which a particular value conflict is resolved can have important implications for future similar situations. Frequent recurrence of specific value conflicts also points to the need for policy recommendations and the formulation of professional standards and position statements to address such conflicts (Dierckx de Casterle 1998).

Taking ethical action

Nurses are encouraged to think about the preferred future they would like for the ethical practice of nursing in the different cultural contexts of the world and to take action to achieve that future (ICN 1999). Thinking about a future ethical world requires vision, moral imagination, critical thinking and intuition, as well as a knowledge of ethics. Doing so allows the nurse to project ethical aspirations about nursing practice excellence and patient care quality into a future that can be reasonably attained. By observing trends in the types of ethical conflicts experienced in practice, nurses can also prepare themselves to respond ethically to these trends which often represent new challenges.

Summary

Nurses may find an ethical decision making model useful in guiding the correct identification, analysis and resolution of ethical issues in nursing practice, and in specific patient care situations. Many such models are available in the nursing literature and many seem to follow a systematic, problem-solving approach to the resolution of value conflicts. Some models represent a traditional, principle-oriented approach to the resolution of value conflicts. In contrast, the model presented here, the Model for Ethical Analysis and Decision Making in Nursing Practice, uses a values-centred approach to the resolution of ethical conflicts in patient care. Because most ethical problems confronting the nurse involve conflicts of values, this model offers a useful approach to analysing ethical issues and making ethical decisions in patient care situations. It can be used alone or in conjunction with other models, depending on the situation.

All nurses should be familiar with theoretically sound ethical decision making models and the ethical approaches they represent. By using a systematic approach to ethical decision making, nurses will maximise both their strategic positions and professional abilities to identify correctly moral problems in the workplace. They will also be able to initiate appropriate and effective strategies to resolve such problems. This, in turn, will help achieve desirable moral outcomes for patients and their caregivers. The consistent demonstration of effective ethical decision making in work-related contexts will establish respect for the nurse as a knowledgeable and skilful person who can assist in the resolution of ethical issues related to patient care.

This guidebook has two foci:

(1) The ICN *Code of Ethics for Nurses* (2006)
(2) The Model for Ethical Analysis and Decision Making in Nursing Practice

The case examples in the chapters that follow include exercises for using the model and applying the ICN *Code of Ethics for Nurses* (2006) to specific patient care situations.

References

Baggs, J.G., Schmitt, M.H., Mushlin, A.I., Eldredge, D.H., Oakes, D. & Hutson, A.D. (1997) Nurse–physician collaboration and satisfaction with the decision-making process in three critical care units. *Amer J Crit Care* 6(5), 393–399.

Berggren, I., Barbosa da Silva, A. & Severinsson, E. (2005) Core ethical issues of clinical nursing supervision. *Nurs Health Sci* 7(1), 21–28.

Davis, A.J., Aroskar, M.A., Liaschenko, J. & Drought, T.S. (1997) *Ethical dilemmas and nursing practice*, 4th ed. Stamford, CT: Appleton & Lange.

Dierckx de Casterle, B. (1998) Supporting nurses in ethical decision making. *Nurs Clin North Am* 33(3), 543–555.

Easen, P. & Wilcockson, J. (1996) Intuition and rational decision-making in professional thinking: A false dichotomy? *J Adv Nurs* 24, 667–673.

Fry, S.T. (2004) Nursing ethics. In S.G. Post (Ed) *Encyclopedia of bioethics*, 3rd ed (pp. 1898–1903). New York: Macmillian Reference USA, Thomson/Gale.

International Council of Nurses (ICN) (1999) *Guidebook for nursing futurists: Future oriented planning for individuals, groups, and associations.* Geneva: ICN.

International Council of Nurses (ICN) (2006) *Code of ethics for nurses.* Geneva: ICN.

Johns, C. (1999) Unravelling the dilemmas within everyday nursing practice. *Nurs Ethics* 6(4), 287–298.

Johnstone, M. (1998) *Determining and responding effectively to ethical professional misconduct: A report to the Nurses Board of Victoria.* Melbourne.

Johnstone, M. (2004) *Bioethics: A nursing perspective*, 3rd ed. Sydney: Harcourt Saunders.

Mariano, C. (2001) Holistic ethics. *ANJ* 101(1), 24A–24C.

Mattison, M. (2000) Ethical decision making: The person in the process. *Social Work* 45(3), 201–212.

Maynard, C.A. (1996) Relationship of critical thinking ability to professional nursing competence. *J Nurs Educ* 35(1), 12–18.

Oddi, L.R., Cassidy, V.R. & Fisher, C. (1995) Nurses' sensitivity to the ethical aspects of clinical practice. *Nurs Ethics* 2(3), 197–209.

Otto, S. & Kennedy-Schwarz (2000) A nurse's lifeline. *AJN* 100(12), 57–59.

Raines, M.L. (2000) Ethical decision making in nurses. Relationships among moral reasoning, coping style, and ethics stress. *JONAS Healthc Law Ethics Regul* 2(1), 29–41.

Rhodes, D. (2000) Pondering an ethical dilemma. *Kai Tiaki Nurs NZ* February, 12–13.

Scott, P.A. (1997) Imagination in practice. *J Med Ethics* 23, 45–50.

Shelly, J.A. (2000) *Spiritual care: A guide for caregivers.* Downer's Grove, IL: Intervarsity Press.

Woods, M. (1999) A nursing ethic: The moral voice of experienced nurses. *Nurs Ethics* 6(5), 423–433.

Yeo, M. & Moorhouse, A. (1996) *Concepts and cases in nursing ethics*, 2nd ed. Ontario, Canada: Broadview Press.

Part 2
Ethical responsibilities of the nurse

The International Council of Nurses (ICN) *Code of Ethics for Nurses* (2006) indicates that nurses have four fundamental responsibilities:

- to promote health
- to prevent illness
- to restore health
- to alleviate suffering

In carrying out these responsibilities, nurses are expected to render healthcare services to individuals, families, groups and the community. They must also co-ordinate their services with the services of other health workers. In promoting health, preventing illness, restoring health and alleviating suffering, the nurse may experience ethical conflict. The nurse must then apply his or her reasoning abilities and ethics knowledge to the patient care situation to determine what action ought to be undertaken.

As discussed in Chapter 5, the use of an ethical decision making model can be helpful to this process. Generally, however, each situation includes elements that make it unique, requiring the nurse to re-examine his or her understanding of nursing responsibilities in light of the specific ethical issues involved. Part 2 will explore the various components of the fundamental responsibilities of the nurse as outlined in the ICN *Code of Ethics for Nurses* (2006). The responsibility to promote health will be analysed in Chapter 6. Other chapters will analyse the nurse's responsibility to prevent illness (Chapter 7), to restore health (Chapter 8) and to alleviate suffering (Chapter 9). Case examples will be used to demonstrate the ethical dimensions of the prescribed four nursing responsibilities in a variety of patient care situations. The Model for Ethical Analysis and Decision Making in Nursing Practice will be used to guide nurses' deliberations on which ethical actions they should take in these situations.

Chapter 6
Promoting health

The nurse's responsibility to promote health is related to the basic right to health long recognised as one of the basic human rights of every person. When introducing the Public Health Act of 1875 to the British Parliament, Prime Minister Disraeli noted that 'the health of the people is really the foundation upon which all their happiness and all their powers of state depend' (Brockington 1956, p. 47).

The right to health is recognised by implementing such public health measures as sanitation and water supply regulations to control the spread of disease. These measures protect the right not to have one's health endangered by the actions of others. Governments recognise this right by enacting laws to prevent the actions of some persons from impairing the health of other persons. All societies expect their leaders and governing bodies to initiate and enforce these laws to promote the health of individuals and society at large (WHO 2002).

Other rights enable citizens to obtain certain healthcare services or community resources. For example, government sponsored programmes of childhood immunisations, food provision, medical care, even education and housing recognise children's rights to health. A pregnant woman's right to health may be protected by subsidised programmes for prenatal care, labour and delivery care and even postpartum care.

Support for a right to health can be found in such documents as the World Health Organization's definition of health which states that '. . . health is one of the fundamental rights of every human being . . .' (World Health Organization 1946) and the Universal Declaration of Human Rights of the United Nations Assembly which notes the right of all persons 'to food, clothing, housing, and medical care' (UNESCO 1949).

The right to healthcare is a right to goods and services that will maintain or improve an individual's existing state of health (Powers & Faden 2006; Teays & Purdy 2001; WHO 2002). It claims that the state or its agencies must provide specific health services that individuals request or are entitled to receive. These services may range from child care and immunisations to home healthcare, nursing homes for the elderly and, in more developed countries, to such costly, high tech, sophisticated procedures as kidney dialysis and organ transplants. The costs of such services are considered, particularly when the individual's right to healthcare conflicts with society's ability to support costly procedures. Nurses often have roles as policy makers helping to establish healthcare priorities, but may experience ethical conflict over which priorities to support. Chapter 7 includes a case example reflecting this conflict (see Case example 9).

Nurses promote the right to health and the right to healthcare by promoting the health of individuals and groups. The ICN Position Statement *Nurses and Human Rights* (2006b) indicates that nurses are primary advocates of the rights of all people to health and healthcare services. Nursing responsibility to promote the health of individuals, groups and communities, is built upon the ethical concept of advocacy. Health-promoting actions by the nurse are clearly supported by the ethical principles of autonomy (the duty to respect self-determined choices), and beneficence and nonmaleficence (the duties to do good and avoid harm). However, ethical issues often arise when carrying out these responsibilities. The following case examples demonstrate situations involving value conflicts that some nurses have experienced while trying to promote health.

Case example 4: Should the nurse give the patient contraceptive information?[1]

What is the story behind the value conflicts?

Ms Hernandez, a public health nurse, recently visited the home of a 24-year-old woman following the birth of her sixth child. Because of her religious beliefs, the young mother practised only natural methods of birth control. However, due to great discomfort and fatigue during the most recent pregnancy, and the needs of her other children, she told Ms Hernandez that she did not want to risk having more children, at least not during the next year or so. She asked how she could obtain information about birth control methods. Ms Hernandez discussed various contraceptive measures available and wrote down the addresses of several family planning clinics near the patient's home. She urged the patient to visit one of the clinics and to select a contraceptive appropriate to her situation.

A few weeks later the patient visited her physician, whose religious beliefs were the same as hers, and told him of her discussion with the nurse and her desire not to have any more children. The physician did not support his patient's interest in contraceptive methods. He later called the nurse's supervisor and told her that he did not want the agency's nurses to engage in any discussions about contraceptives with his patients. He did not think it was a nurse's business to discuss family planning with patients, especially when the patient's religious beliefs prohibited the use of birth control methods.

Ms Hernandez thought that withholding contraception information to patients who request the information was a violation of her duty toward them. But she did not want to take any action that could potentially harm her patients. What should she do?

What is the significance of the values involved?

This case example shows how the nurse's responsibility to promote health can be constrained by religious beliefs held by the patient and/or other health workers. Where family planning questions are concerned, nurses must consider their own personal beliefs, their country's official government policy on family planning, and the scope of the responsibility to promote health. However, it is known that lower birth rates are positively correlated with improved maternal and child health, reduced infant mortality, and increased opportunities for women in many countries (Boston Women's Health Book Collective 2005).

Nurses are expected to value professional standards and health regulations that promote the health of individuals. Such values may also contribute significantly to the health of families and communities. Patients, however, may place greater value on their religious beliefs and the practices supported by their culture and not on the values represented by healthcare agencies and health professionals. Providing information about artificial methods of contraception to a young woman who values her health and ability to care for existing children as well as her religious and cultural values may lead to a conflict of values that can be difficult to resolve.

In such situations, nurses play important roles as patient advocates. By supporting the patient's values and choices, they advocate the basic human rights of individuals to be respected as independent decision makers in control of their own destinies. As a patient advocate, the nurse also supports the health and the well-being of the patient as defined by the patient and not someone else (Fry & Veatch 2006; Schoen 2005). This is part of the nurse's fundamental responsibility to promote health.

What is the significance of the conflicts to the parties involved?

Providing contraceptive information to a woman who requests it and whose health suggests a need to refrain from childbearing seems necessary if one takes seriously the nurse's fundamental responsibility to promote health (ICN 2006a). But should the nurse do so if the information requested conflicts with the patient's religious beliefs? Should the nurse do so when the patient's physician asks that the nurse not provide such information?

As a nurse, Ms Hernandez should be concerned about the overall health of this patient and the six children she has borne in a relatively short time (ICN 2002). A decline in the mother's health could well affect her ability to care for the new infant and her other children. The mother's request for information about artificial methods of contraception as a means to promote her health cannot be ignored by the nurse. The nurse is primarily responsible to the patient, and secondarily to the physician and the nursing agency.

The presence of value conflict is not a situation to be avoided, but may be an opportunity for the nurse to share valuable information with patients, to engage in health teaching and to assist patients to make health choices consistent with their values. By open discussion with this patient, the nurse can encourage her to examine her values and the basis of her desire not to bear another child in the near future. The patient can also be encouraged to discuss these wishes with her partner, and her religious advisor, if possible. By examining all the options open to her, the young mother will be able to understand the consequences of any judgments and choices she might make related to childbearing. Whether she decides to seek or not seek contraceptive advice, the young mother will know that she is making an informed decision, knowing all options and their potential results, and is supported in her decision by the nurse.

What should be done?

Presuming that Ms Hernandez's religious beliefs do not conflict with providing contraceptive information and that family planning is encouraged by her country's health policies, the nurse should provide the requested contraceptive information to this patient and any other patient. By discussing the uses and availability of various contraceptives, the patient can learn about the options open to her. By encouraging the patient to discuss her family situation and how she makes important decisions in other areas of her life, the nurse can learn more about this patient's value system. The nurse's interest in the woman's health and the respectful consideration of her values will help the patient weigh the importance of her religious beliefs against her need to refrain from bearing children (Schoen 2005). The nurse should do whatever she can to promote the health of this patient while respecting the right of the patient to choose the course of action most appropriate to her own situation.

Some countries do not have a policy that promotes family planning as a means to improve maternal and child health. In these countries, the nurse should do whatever she can to document how the lack of family planning services affects the health of individuals and families, especially the health of women and children. Through their national nursing association, nurses can propose changes in government policy on family planning and assist in the development of specific programmes. They can also discuss family planning issues with other nurses and physicians in local and national forums. Such discussion will help guide individual nurses when these issues arise and will help reconceptualise nursing practice and the scope of nurses' responsibilities and commitments to achieve health for all (Aroskar 1995).

Case example 5: When promoting health means to choose among patients[2]

What is the story behind the value conflicts?

Ines Aguinaga, the night nurse, reviews the needs of her patients on a small medical-surgical nursing care unit. Mrs R is an 83-year-old woman who has had a stroke and is expected to die. She is semicomatose and needs suctioning every 15 to 20 minutes. Mr J is a 47-year-old man admitted this afternoon for observation following the passage of several bloody stools. His vital signs are stable but he is complaining of severe abdominal pain. Mr P, a 52-year-old man recently diagnosed with diabetes, has unstable blood sugar levels and is receiving intravenous insulin. His urinary output has been very low and he is having wide blood pressure swings. Ms M is a 35-year-old patient who learned today that she has ovarian cancer with metastasis to the pelvis and spine. She has a history of suicidal attempts and is experiencing severe pain. Six other patients are recovering from surgical procedures and are considered stable. Which patients should be the highest priority to receive nursing care from Ms Aguinaga? Is it ethical to promote the health of one patient over that of another?

What is the significance of the values involved?

Nurses usually have responsibility for the care of several patients at one time and are obliged to promote the health and well-being of all patients. Yet, it may be physically impossible for a nurse to promote the health and well-being of all patients at the same time. The nurse must choose which patient should receive nursing attention first while trying to ensure their choice does not harm other patients who must wait. How the nurse makes that choice reflects an assessment of patient needs, a knowledge of illness states, and careful judgment of how to promote health as an ethical responsibility (Fry & Veatch 2006).

Ms Aguinaga knows that she is obliged to promote the health of each of her patients and that she can promote health by providing certain benefits to them. The problem is that she has ten patients, each of whom requires her care and can conceivably benefit from it. However, it would be physically impossible to provide full benefits to all patients at the same time, and it is apparent that four patients are in greater need of nursing attention than the rest.

What is the significance of the conflicts to the parties involved?

Ms Aguinaga might decide to give equal amounts of attention to each of the four patients, but this would not promote the health of these patients equally. Each patient has different needs for nursing care and each will receive varying degrees of benefit from her nursing care.

She could attempt to determine where she can promote the health of one patient to its fullest extent and begin with that patient. Making this kind of decision will be subjective, however, and will force her to decide whether it is most beneficial to:

(1) suction an inevitably dying patient
(2) prevent insulin shock
(3) monitor internal bleeding
(4) prevent plans for suicide in a patient suffering from the end stages of a cancer-related illness

Though some patients might receive more short-term health benefit from receiving her attention first (Mrs R, for example, will not have her breathing impaired) it remains unclear where the greatest amount of long-term benefit can be achieved by choosing one patient over another for primary attention.

She could make a decision that the age of the patient is related to health benefit. In that case, the youngest patient (Ms M) surely would have the highest priority for Ms Aguinaga. But who is to say that the health of the youngest patient is more important than the health of any older patient? The youngest patient might argue that receiving benefit at an earlier age contributes to cumulative benefits over a lifetime; hence, the nurse would be obliged to serve the youngest patients first. But should age be a deciding factor in the promotion of health and is cumulative health promotion the goal of the nurse?

If the needs of all patients are considered, the patient with the greatest need might realise the greatest benefit but that is not certain. If the suffering of a patient helps the nurse to determine whom to care for first, then perhaps Mrs R should be the first priority since she will undoubtedly suffer if not suctioned. If reduction of suffering is considered the greatest benefit for a patient, then this should be the action to follow. It is important to point out, however, that promoting health cannot be equated with providing the greatest benefit to patients. Promoting the health of patients is a specific moral task of the nurse and cannot be reduced to the mere promotion of overall good or individual patient benefit (Fry & Veatch 2006).

What should be done?

To many people, the decision faced by Ms Aguinaga is one that simply requires nursing competence and managerial experience. They might argue that the competent nurse will 'know' what to do in this type of situation. The competent nurse will make a decision that constitutes safe and prudent nursing care and will promote health by providing this level of care. Deciding what to do merely reflects Ms Aguinaga's decision-making skill and clinical competence.

However, because the promotion of health is an ethical responsibility of the nurse, the ethical dimensions of this situation cannot be easily dismissed. Nurses make ethical decisions that promote health. The decisions are based on the nurse's judgment about what is ethically required and not merely what is most efficient in managing patients and their needs. To promote health is to make an ethical judgment of what is required of the nurse. The ability to make an ethical judgment may not correlate to a nurse's clinical or managerial competence. One can make an efficient managerial decision that is morally wrong. It would be morally wrong if the rights of the patients were not respected, for example.

Ms Aguinaga needs to determine what is required to promote the immediate health and well-being of the patients under her care. If Mrs R will suffocate from not being suctioned, then her immediate health and well-being require that she be given nursing attention before anything else. Mrs R's needs will continue to take priority in the nurse's health promotion activities.

Ms M's pain and risk of suicide can be an immediate threat to her health and well-being, thus Ms Aguinaga needs to attend to her needs next. Once the immediate needs of these two patients are addressed and their conditions stabilised, the nurse can determine how best to observe and monitor the health needs of Mr J and Mr P. If the condition of either or both changes so as to warrant the nurse's full attention, this attention can now be given with the knowledge that the health and well-being of the other two patients will not be seriously compromised. Promoting the health and well-being of patients often requires more from the nurse than an assessment of the benefits and harms of specific nursing care in patient populations. It requires the nurse to make an ethical judgment about how the health and well-being of patients can be best promoted through nursing care.

The responsibility to promote health may involve discussions with patients about genetic testing. Awareness of genetically related illnesses has increased throughout the world. This awareness has resulted, in part, from the significant progress of researchers in mapping the approximately 100 000 genes located within the cells of the human body (Jenkins, Grady & Collins 2005). Genetic knowledge will ultimately make it possible to diagnose and treat many diseases that were not well understood or treatable. Genetic testing (which involves DNA analysis), in particular, identifies an individual's risk of being a carrier of a disease or the risk of bearing a child with a genetically related disorder. Pre-symptomatic testing identifies whether a person has a gene for a specific disease but does not have signs or symptoms of the disease. Susceptibility testing identifies genes that are associated with specific illnesses, such as breast cancer or Alzheimer's disease (Collins & Barker 2007; Scanlon & Fibison 1995; Williams 2000). The following case example demonstrates ethical issues that arise in the care of a patient who is considering genetic testing.

Case example 6: The patient who undergoes genetic testing

What is the story behind the value conflicts?

Terese' D is a genetics nurse in a genetics testing clinic in a large city. Today, she is expecting Mrs G, a 38-year-old woman, to return to the clinic for a report on genetic testing she had two weeks ago. Mrs G's physician wanted her to undergo genetic testing because she has very high blood lipid levels (hyperlipidemia) and there is a significant history of heart disease in her family. The testing will confirm whether or not she has a genetic predisposition to familial heart disease and her current condition of hyperlipidemia. If she does, knowing this genetic component of her condition will be useful to designing a treatment plan for Mrs G.

In reviewing the results of Mrs G's genetics testing, Terese' D discovers that this patient not only has the genetic alteration consistent with familial heart disease (which explains, in part, her hyperlipidemia), but also has a double dose of this genetic alteration, which is found in only a very small percentage of the population. Unfortunately, a double dose of this particular gene is associated with the onset of Alzheimer's disease. What should Terese' D do with this information? Should she tell Mrs G about this unintended result of the testing?

What is the significance of the values involved?

Mrs G has already indicated that genetic information is of significant value to her and her quality of life. She wants to know whether she is genetically predisposed to familial heart disease as this will influence her treatment, especially medication, and probably her lifestyle, in terms of diet and exercise. Since she already values this information, it is likely that she would value knowing that she is pre-disposed to Alzheimer's disease, as well. However, if the potential of finding unintended information as a result of the genetics testing was not discussed with her prior to testing, it is not certain that she wants to know this information.

Terese' D, as a nurse, values being truthful with her patients and might believe that any patient has a moral right to information about themselves, especially genetic information which is the most fundamental and private information a person can have. However, Mrs G did not know that additional information that could affect her health might be discovered by the genetic test. The information that Mrs G is susceptible to the development of Alzheimer's disease might be more information than she can reasonably handle at the present time and might be psychologically harmful to her.

What is the significance of the conflicts to the parties involved?

Nurses have an obligation to be truthful in their care of patients and should not withhold information from them, especially information that might affect their health. The nurse has a responsibility to promote health which means to discuss anything with a patient that might affect the patient's health status (ICN 2006a).

Known susceptibility to Alzheimer's disease is a morally and materially significant piece of information. Currently there is no cure for the disease. An accelerated death of brain cells, loss of memory and loss of the ability to function independently are the grim hallmarks. If Mrs G had one gene that predisposed her to the disease, that would mean that she had about a 45% chance of developing the disease by age 80 (Nussbaum, McInnes & Willard 2007). However, she has two genes that predispose her to the disease giving her a 90% risk of developing the disease. This predisposition to the disease is quite substantial. This does not mean that it is certain that she will develop the disease. Even those without the gene have a 20% possibility of developing the disease in later life. The development of Alzheimer's disease is known to be affected by environmental factors, such as diet and blows to the head, as well as exposure to toxins or infections. Genetics predisposition is just one part of the total picture. The genetic predisposition has been with Mrs G since conception and concerns the way the gene carries out its function in the cell (Nussbaum, McInnes & Willard 2007). However, there is no known cure for the disease and, at best, treatment can only slow down the development of the disease.

Terese' D knows this information and thinks that Mrs G should know this information, as well. But she does not want to cause harm to Mrs G by providing her with information that could have psychological and emotional impact (Fleming 2002). Should she tell Mrs G the full results of her genetic testing?

What should be done?

To resolve the conflict, Terese' D should first find out whether Mrs G wants to know all information gained from the genetic testing. Ideally, this should have been discussed prior to testing and Mrs G should have indicated her willingness, in writing, to receive all information. Most genetic clinics have policies to cover this kind of situation and to clarify what the role of the genetics nurse should be in disclosing the unintended results of testing to patients (Scanlon & Fibison 1995).

Second, the nurse should have knowledge of potential treatments for Mrs G's condition and be able to refer her to resources for those treatments. In the case of Alzheimer's disease, this is especially important because there are probably changes that Mrs G can make in her diet and medications that she can take that are known to delay the onset of the disease. The nurse also has a responsibility to prevent illness, whenever the nurse can do so (ICN 2006a).

Last, Terese' D should participate in her clinic's development of policies and written agreements with patients that will protect the rights of patients to decide the information they want known about themselves, through genetic testing, and what information they want disclosed to them from genetic testing. All nurses who care for patients receiving the results of genetic testing should participate in the development of these policies as a part of their advocacy role in patient care. Providing genetic information to patients can significantly influence their quality of life and future health status.

Exercise:

> **Case example 7: When an inexperienced nurse is assigned to a rural clinic**
>
> *What is the story behind the value conflicts?*
>
> A young nurse midwife, Ms Mbabali, has been directed to accompany a physician going to a rural clinic served by the district hospital. The nurse has had little unsupervised practice experience. The nurse supervisor believes that the 4-day visit to the clinic will provide valuable experience for the young nurse. The physician promises to be available for necessary supervision and guidance.
>
> During the clinic visit, several difficult births occur. While the physician is performing an unexpected Caesarean birth (the second in 12 hours), Ms Mbabali and the regular clinic nurse supervise the labour and birthing of several other women.
>
> The first birthing is normal, Ms Mbabali experiences no difficulty, and the mother and child continue to do well. The second birthing is more difficult. The woman, who is HIV-positive, simply appears at the clinic in strong labour, riding in the back of a van. The birthing is complicated and the infant dies following its birth. No family members are present and the woman has been gravely ill since the delivery.
>
> Ms Mbabali has some misgivings about her performance in managing the labour and birthing of this woman. The physician was in surgery at that time and the regular clinic nurse was visiting mothers and children at a nearby village. She wonders whether she did all that was appropriate for the health of the mother and the welfare of the infant.
>
> Now, a third woman is presenting with a difficult labour and Ms Mbabali wants closer supervision by the physician or the regular clinic nurse, both of whom are occupied with other patients. The regular clinic nurse is upset because she expects Ms Mbabali to know more about difficult births than she is able to demonstrate. The physician is clearly not pleased that she lacks confidence in her ability with this birthing but he encourages her, telling her to do her best.
>
> The nurse midwife wonders whether she may have contracted the HIV virus from the second woman. She is concerned about her ability to bring the mother and child through the present labour and birthing without incident. She is worried that she might not pass her forthcoming certification exam. She is also worried about what the physician and regular clinic nurse will tell her nursing supervisor when she returns from the field experience. What should she do?

Discussion questions

What is the story behind the value conflicts?

(1) What are the problems as defined by Ms Mbabali? By the physician? By the regular clinic nurse? By the HIV-positive woman? By the woman currently in labour?

(2) What values are involved from each person's view?

What is the significance of the values involved?

(3) What are the meanings of these values to each person involved? What does it mean for the nurse to promote health in this situation?

(4) Are there any legal or professional practice questions involved in this situation?

(5) Which values seem to conflict with others?

What is the significance of the conflicts to the parties involved?

(6) Which value conflicts are the most significant to the individuals involved?

(7) How might the value conflicts affect Ms Mbabali's nursing practice?

(8) How might the value conflicts affect the woman who is in labour and under Ms Mbabali's care? How might these conflicts lead to policy formation?

(9) Should an inexperienced nurse be held accountable for promoting the health of patients to the same extent as a more experienced nurse? Why or why not?

(10) Does promoting the health of patients require the nurse to put her own health at risk when no other form of healthcare is available for the patient? Does promoting the health of patients mean the nurse's health is secondary to patient health and well-being?

(11) If Ms Mbabali should contract HIV infection, who is responsible for this?

What should be done?

(12) What are the possible ways to resolve the value conflicts in this situation?

(13) What are the probable outcomes of these resolutions?

(14) What actions should Ms Mbabali follow in this situation? Why?

(15) How could these value conflicts be prevented in the future?

Summary

Nurses carry out a fundamental responsibility to the patient when they promote health. This is an ethical responsibility that takes on additional meaning within the context of specific patient care situations (Romyn 2003). Providing contraceptive information to a patient whose religious beliefs forbid their use tests the meaning of promoting health. Likewise, deciding how to allocate one's time and attention among needy patients tests the relevance of ethical principles as guides to nursing actions. Sending an inexperienced nurse to provide needed nursing care in a remote rural area tests the meaning of health promotion. However, in situations where resources are limited, care provided by even inexperienced nurses might be better than no care at all (Shallat 1990). In these situations, nurses must balance their responsibility to provide good with their responsibility to prevent and reduce risks of harm.

The ethical responsibility to promote health is not the same as the ethical responsibility to provide benefit to patients. The ethical dimensions of the latter responsibility cannot be reduced to a mere calculation of harms and benefits provided by nursing care. Likewise, the promotion of health requires the nurse to make an ethical judgment about the measures required for each patient's health. Each patient situation has cultural, social and political dimensions that make the nurse's ethical responsibility to promote health a challenging endeavour.

Notes

1 Adapted from Tate, B.L. (1977) *The nurse's dilemma: Ethical considerations in nursing practice.* Geneva: ICN (p. 18). Used with permission.
2 Adapted from Fry, S.T. & Veatch, R.M. (2006) *Case studies in nursing ethics*, 3rd ed. Boston: Jones & Bartlett (pp. 99–101). Used with permission.

References

Aroskar, M.A. (1995) Envisioning nursing as a moral community. *Nurs Outlook* 43(3), 134–138.

Beauchamp, D. & Steinbock, B. (1999) *New ethics for the public's health.* New York: Oxford University Press.

Boston Women's Health Book Collective (2005) *Our bodies, ourselves: A new edition for a new era.* New York: Simon & Schuster.

Brockington, C. (1956) *A short history of public health.* London: Churchill.

Collins, F. & Barker, A.D. (2007) Mapping the cancer genome: Pinpointing the gene involved in cancer will help chart a new course across the complex landscape of human malignancies. *Sci Am* 296(3), 50–57.

Fleming, D.A. (2002) Ethical considerations of genetic testing. *J Clin Ethics* 13(4), 316–323.

Fry, S.T. & Veatch, R.M. (2006) *Case studies in nursing ethics*, 3rd ed. Boston: Jones & Bartlett, Publishers.

International Council of Nurses (ICN) (2002) *Position statement: Women's health.* Geneva, Switzerland: ICN.

International Council of Nurses (ICN) (2006a) *Code of ethics for nurses.* Geneva, Switzerland: ICN.

International Council of Nurses (ICN) (2006b) *Position statement: Nurses and human rights.* Geneva, Switzerland: ICN.

Jenkins, J., Grady, P.A. & Collins, F.S. (2005) Nurses and the genome revolution. *J Nurs Scholarship* 37(3), 98–101.

Nussbaum, R.L., McInnes, R.R. & Willard, H.F. (2007) *Genetics in medicine.* Philadelphia: Elsevier Health Sciences.

Powers, M. & Faden, R. (2006) *Social justice: The moral foundations of public health and health policy.* New York: Oxford University Press.

Romyn, D.M. (2003) The relational narrative: Implications for nurse practice and education. *Nurs Philos* 4(2), 149–154.

Scanlon, D. & Fibison, W. (1995) *Managing genetic information: Implications for nursing practice.* Washington, DC: American Nurses Association.

Schoen, J. (2005) *Choice and coercion: Birth control, sterilization, and abortion in public health and welfare.* Chapel Hill, NC: University of North Carolina Press.

Shallat, L. (1990) Women and AIDS: The unprotected sex. *Wom Hlth J* 18, 26–49.

Teays, W. & Purdy, L. (Eds) (2001) *Bioethics, justice, & health care*. Belmont, CA: Wadsworth/Thomson Learning.

UNESCO (1949) *Human rights: A symposium*. New York: Allan Wingate.

Williams, J.K. (2000) Impact of genome research on children and their families. *J Ped Nurs* 15(4), 207–211.

World Health Organization (WHO) (1946) Constitution of the World Health Organization. *Off Rec Wld Hlth Org*, 2, 100.

World Health Organization (WHO) (2002) *25 Questions & answers on health & human rights*. Health & Human Rights Publication Series, Issue No.1. Geneva: WHO.

Chapter 7
Preventing illness

All people have the right to the highest attainable standard of health (CESCR 2000). Supported by various international instruments (covenants, conventions and treaties), the right to health has been authoritatively interpreted as entailing a claim to 'a set of social arrangements – norms, institutions, laws, an enabling environment – that can best secure the enjoyment of this right' (WHO 2002, pp. 8, 9 & 11).

All health professionals working in countries that are signatories to the international instruments supporting the right to health have a stringent responsibility to support the development and implementation of 'social arrangements' that secure the right to health of individuals, families and communities. This responsibility extends to also supporting processes designed to reduce the incidence and negative impact of otherwise preventable illness.

The ICN has identified 'preventing illness' as one of four fundamental responsibilities of the nurse. This responsibility is underpinned by the principles and standards of human rights (ICN 2006a) and by the ethical values and concepts (e.g. advocacy and caring) contained in the ICN (2006b) *Code of Ethics for Nurses*. As with promoting health, the responsibility to prevent illness is also supported by the broader bioethical principles of beneficence, nonmaleficence and justice, and the related obligations on the part of caregivers to prevent or avoid harm.

In promoting health, however, as well as upholding other duties, nurses are obliged to also support 'necessary safeguards to protect the privacy of patient records' (ICN 2000). In keeping with this obligation, nurses have a responsibility to ensure they are familiar with the 'rights, responsibilities, protocols and legislation in their country, regarding patients' rights to privacy' (ICN 2000). Professional nursing associations, meanwhile, 'should assist nurses in understanding and exercising their responsibilities' in regard to protecting a patient's health information – including their right to have access to that information (ICN 2000).

In accordance with both the philosophy and ethical standards of the nursing profession, nurses are obliged to reduce the incidence and impact of otherwise preventable harm to people, including the preventable harms that might and do occur as a result of illness. Just how far a nurse can – and should – go in preventing illness, however, is open to question – particularly when the kinds of interventions required may be beyond the capacity of an individual nurse to provide and/or paradoxically may place the nurse at odds with the rights or expressed wishes of a patient, family or community. The following case example illustrates this question in the care of a patient threatened with an incurable disease.

Case example 8: Preventing HIV transmission to an unsuspecting patient[1]

What is the story behind the value conflicts?

Sharon McBride recently accepted a staff nurse position at a weight loss clinic within a large urban hospital. She had previously worked in another hospital serving an inner city population that included injecting drug users, some of whom tested positive for the human immunodeficiency virus (HIV). Distressed by the frequent re-admissions of these patients and the limited success of the treatment programmes being offered, she sought employment that was more related to health promotion rather than acute in-patient care. One of her clinic patients is Anne, a severely overweight 32-year-old divorced mother of two children. Anne was recently diagnosed with a mild heart arrhythmia, high blood pressure and decreased kidney function secondary to repeated episodes of pyelonephritis. Her primary care physician has advised her to lose 16 kilos (40 pounds).

As Anne nears her weight loss goal, she tells Ms McBride that she has a new boyfriend who is planning to move into her apartment. One day, the boyfriend accompanies Anne to her clinic visit. Ms McBride recognises him as a patient that she cared for at the inner city hospital, and remembers that he tested HIV-positive after entering a drug treatment programme. Ms McBride asks Anne about her boyfriend and learns that she knows about his previous injecting drug use, but seems to be unaware that he tested HIV-positive over a year ago. Ms McBride manages to speak to the boyfriend alone and he acknowledges that he was a patient in the other hospital but denies that he ever tested positive for HIV. He tells the nurse that she must have him confused with some other patient. Ms McBride does not think this is the case but is not sure what she can do under the circumstances. One month later, Anne shyly tells Ms McBride that she thinks she is pregnant. Should Ms McBride share her concerns about the boyfriend's possible HIV-positive status with Anne? Should she confirm her suspicions by asking a colleague at the other hospital to look up the result of the HIV/AIDS blood test in the boyfriend's health record? Does she have any obligation to Anne and Anne's boyfriend concerning the transmission of HIV and the prevention of AIDS?

What is the significance of the values involved?

HIV infection is a major health and socio-economic concern throughout the world (Harris & Siplon 2001; Hunt 2004; Poku 2006). HIV can lead to acquired immunodeficiency syndrome (AIDS) in humans, a collection of diseases that has simultaneously emerged as 'a tragedy for individuals, families and communities and a threat to sustainable development' – particularly in developing countries (Poku 2006, p. 346). According to the latest figures published by the UNAIDS/WHO (2006) AIDS epidemic update, an estimated 39.5 million people are living with HIV. Alarmingly, despite the demonstrated success of HIV prevention and treatment services in reducing illness and disease from HIV/AIDS, there were 4.3 million new infections recorded in 2006, with 65% (2.8 million) of these occurring in sub-Saharan Africa. In 2006, 2.9 million people died of AIDS-related illnesses; this figure is projected to increase dramatically in the coming years, with experts suggesting that 'if prevention and vaccine are not on the horizon soon, more than 68 million people will die of the infection in the next two decades' (Hunt 2004, p. 468). The economic and social costs of this mortality rate are predicted to be dire – particularly in developing countries, which are already experiencing an explosive increase in the number of children being orphaned as a result of their parents dying from AIDS; the erosion of their labour forces and the related inability to fill job vacancies; the loss of healthcare professionals, military and peace keeping forces (it has been estimated that in countries with an HIV prevalence rate of 30%, between 3% and 7% of healthcare workers will be lost annually to AIDS (Harris & Siplon 2001, p. 32) – in some countries health worker deaths from HIV has been as high as 17% and projected to increase to a total of 40% by 2010 (WHO 2006a)); and the destruction of 'intergenerational social cultural capital formation' and with it 'the ability of succeeding generations to maintain the development achievements of the past' (Poku 2006, p. 346; see also Hunt 2004).

First identified by French and United States researchers in the early 1980s, HIV may be transmitted by sexual, parenteral and perinatal routes and through an exchange of body fluids with an infected person (Cameron 1993). The virus penetrates the human immune system's CD4 cells that are essential to maintaining the body's defence against infection and disease. Once within these cells, the virus can remain latent for prolonged periods of time (10 years or more) without the infected individual showing any symptoms of infection or illness. Once infected, the HIV-positive person can transmit the virus to others without knowing it. Given the debilitating, potentially fatal effects of AIDS (the disease may or may not cause death, depending on the access a person has to a high standard of living and modern healthcare (Hunt 2004, p. 467)), the prevention of HIV infection is of great concern to governments, citizens, and healthcare workers alike in the world (ICN 2001; UNAIDS/WHO 2006; WHO 2006b).

What is the significance of the conflicts to the parties involved?

Ms McBride has a justifiable ethical concern about the threat of HIV transmission to her patient. She can verify her suspicion that Anne's boyfriend is HIV-positive by obtaining information from his patient record at the other hospital. If she does so, however, she will be engaging in unethical and possibly even illegal behaviour as a nurse. Since she is no longer employed by the first hospital, she does not have authorised access to any information in the boyfriend's healthcare record. Moreover, accessing his healthcare record without his permission could be construed as unethical conduct. This is because accessing the healthcare record without the boyfriend's permission would be an infringement of his right to privacy – specifically, his right to self-determine who will have access to information about him and for what purposes. The threat of HIV transmission, albeit potentially significant, might not justify Ms McBride accessing the boyfriend's healthcare record, even though strong moral reasons could be provided for overriding his right to privacy – bearing in mind that the right to privacy and confidentiality is not absolute and may be overridden by other stronger moral considerations (Johnstone 2004). For instance, if Ms McBride and her boyfriend have engaged in unprotected sex resulting in pregnancy, and continue to do so throughout her pregnancy, there is a quantifiable risk (if indeed her boyfriend is HIV-positive) of both Ms McBride and her unborn child acquiring HIV infection – it would then further need to be weighed up whether this situation justifies breaching his right to privacy by informing Anne of his HIV status.

What should be done?

Should Ms McBride simply tell Anne about her suspicions concerning the new boyfriend? If Ms McBride was to reveal to Anne the information she has about the boyfriend's HIV status, she would be in breach of her professional obligation to protect patient confidentiality, one of the most fundamental obligations of all healthcare workers (Fry & Veatch 2006). Ms McBride is acutely aware, however, that if Anne has contracted HIV from her boyfriend there are significant risks of it being transmitted to her child either in utero or during labour (Foster & Lyall 2005; Kourtis et al. 2001; Ostergren & Malyuta 2006; Petropoulou et al. 2006). She is also aware that there is a strong direct relationship between primary prevention activities and lower infections in infants, and that 'voluntary HIV testing and counselling in general, and particularly during pregnancy, provide an excellent opportunity to address HIV prevention among women and infants' (Ostergren & Malyuta 2006, p. 56; see also Hunt 2004). To carry out her responsibility to prevent illness in Anne, her infant and her family, Ms McBride will thus have to consider other actions.

Ms McBride could use her former relationship with the boyfriend to get him to consider the threat that his (possible) positive HIV status poses to Anne and the child she is carrying. She could advise him that being HIV-positive is not necessarily the 'death sentence' it was once considered to be – provided it is managed responsibly. She could point out that if Anne is infected, the risks of HIV being transmitted to their baby could be dramatically reduced through antiretroviral therapy (ART) during pregnancy, planned pre-labour Caesarean section (usually at 38–39 weeks), and neonatal ART after birth for the first 4–6 weeks of life (Foster & Lyall 2005; Kourtis et al. 2001; Ostergren & Malyuta 2006). Finally, Ms McBride might also need to consider informing the boyfriend that, under local Department of Health guidelines, she is obliged to notify his case to the Department. She could add, however, that although she is legally required to make such a notification, she would prefer to do so with his full knowledge and consent. She could add that, with his permission, she would like to contact and discuss his case with the Department of Health Department Contact Tracers (also called Partner Notification Officers) who are available to give confidential advice on these matters as well as doing the actual contact tracing on behalf of a source person (i.e. the boyfriend in this case).

If the boyfriend is HIV-positive and still refuses to consent to a disclosure being made to his girlfriend, Ms McBride has little option and will have to inform the Contact Tracers who will follow up with Anne (she takes some comfort in knowing that Contact Tracers do not disclose the name to the source person or the name of the person doing the reporting).

Ms McBride could also use her relationship with Anne to explore her understanding of safe sexual practices and educate her about the need to protect herself and her fetus from HIV and other sexually transmissible infections. If she should become HIV-positive, she and her fetus will be at risk of serious HIV-related illness, and her two other children could lose their parent because, without treatment, the disease is frequently fatal. This is arguably one of the most compelling arguments that she can use to encourage Anne to consider full ante-natal screening with pre- and post-HIV test counselling from a clinic with expertise in this area, along with screening for other blood-borne viruses. She could add that, given her boyfriend's past injecting drug use (and the known associated risk of acquiring HIV, HCV (see Zanetti et al. 2006) and other blood-borne viruses), it would be wise to encourage the boyfriend to have an HIV test and to take appropriate actions once the results are known. Ms McBride would not only be morally justified in taking such action, but, as required by the ICN *Code of Ethics for Nurses* (2006b) and related Position Statement on AIDS (ICN 2001), she would also be fulfilling her professional responsibility to prevent illness in this patient, her infant and her family.

Case example 9: Preventing illness while protecting the 'right to decide' and confidentiality of a pregnant young teenage patient

What is the story behind the value conflicts?

Joanne Briganti is working in the intensive care unit (ICU) of a major metropolitan health service located in a poor suburb that also has a high incidence of young teenage pregnancies (pregnancies in teenagers under 15 years of age). Robyn ('Bobbie') Kingston, a 14-year-old female, accompanied by her mother, has been admitted to the ICU in a state of acute respiratory distress following a severe asthma attack The teenager is also suffering from septicaemia as a result of a urinary tract infection that has not responded to a course of antibiotics that she has been taking. Upon being admitted to the ICU, ED staff handing over to the ICU staff confirm that Bobbie has had chest x-rays (which had to be repeated because the first films were not clear), has been commenced on steroids and has been given a bronchial dilator via a nebuliser. The staff also confirm that Bobbie has been started on intravenous antibiotics for her urinary tract infection.

During the admission procedure, Ms Briganti thinks that Bobbie 'looks' pregnant. There is, however, no indication in the teenager's ED admission record that she is pregnant. When Ms Briganti examines the teenager's hospital notes containing details of her previous admissions (which have just been delivered to the ICU) she discovers a record indicating that Bobbie has had two abortions over the past 12 months. Ms Briganti is not sure what to do. She is mindful that treating Bobbie's asthma and getting her stabilised is the primary concern of the healthcare team at the moment. Not knowing whether the teenager is pregnant, however, is problematic since, if Bobbie is pregnant, this will need to be taken into consideration in the planning and delivery of her medical treatment and nursing care. Ms Briganti is particularly concerned that if she asks the teenager whether she is pregnant, this might cause her added distress. On the other hand, by not knowing whether Bobbie is pregnant, appropriate care (including making a referral to the hospital's social worker) cannot be initiated.

Bobbie is extremely ill. She is labouring to breathe and there are clinical signs suggesting that her septicaemia is worsening. Should Ms Briganti ask Bobbie if she is pregnant? Should she ask the doctors managing Bobbie's case to order a pregnancy test 'without Bobbie knowing about it'? Should Ms Briganti ask Bobbie's mother whether the teenager is pregnant? Should the hospital's social worker be called in regardless?

What is the significance of the values involved?

Healthcare professionals have a stringent responsibility for initiating and supporting actions aimed at ensuring that people's health and care needs are met. The ICN *Code of Ethics for Nurses* contains provisions clarifying that 'nurses share with society the responsibility for initiating and supporting action to meet the health and social needs of the public, in particular those of vulnerable populations' (ICN 2006b, p. 2). In fulfilling this responsibility, however, health professionals (including nurses) also have a duty to ensure that people are enabled to make informed choices about their care and treatment. In response to this requirement, the ICN *Code of Ethics for Nurses* prescribes, 'The nurse ensures that the individual receives sufficient information on which to base consent for care and related treatment' (ICN 2006b, p. 2). Taking into account people's entitlements to and in healthcare are to be 'unrestricted by considerations of age', this means that even those below a legal consenting age (e.g. 'mature minors') are entitled, where able, to participate in decision making concerning their care and treatment (Cook & Dickens 2000; Derish & Vanden Heuvel 2000; Dickens & Cook 2005).

Another important requirement is that healthcare professionals keep in confidence information gained in the context of the professional–patient relationship (Fry & Veatch 2006; Johnstone 2004). Almost all codes of healthcare ethics contain provisions concerning confidentiality, including the ICN *Code of Ethics for Nurses* (2006b). Ethical reasons to maintain confidentiality include protecting the patient from the harms that can occur as a result of disclosures being made without consent, and protecting the trust and integrity that is inherent in the nurse–patient relationship. Maintaining confidentiality is also supported by a principle of privacy and the right of the patient to determine what personal information will be known by others, under what circumstances, and for what reasons.

Because of a general right to privacy, health professionals are obligated to keep information disclosed in professional–patient relationships private and confidential. Thus, when overriding circumstances arise that may require confidential information gained in a professional–patient relationship to be disclosed to another appropriate person, the nurse must not only 'use careful judgment in sharing this information' (ICN 2006b, p. 2), but must also be able to provide a sound moral justification – that is, the 'strongest moral reasons' – for doing so (Johnstone 2004, pp. 35–36). The issue of confidential healthcare for adolescents (defined by WHO as being between the ages of 10 and 19 years) has become the subject of much debate in recent years, as young people's 'sexual and reproductive health rights' have been brought increasingly into focus in the public arena and confronting questions raised about the rights of parents to override the independent choices and judgments made by their adolescent children (Cook & Dickens 2000; Dickens & Cook 2005; Lehrer et al. 2007; Sanci et al. 2005; Sundby 2006).

Thus, sharing information with appropriate adults (e.g. parents) in the case of teenage pregnancies may not be as strongly warranted as it might at first appear to be – there may, for instance, be strong moral reasons for not disclosing confidential information about a young teenager's pregnancy to a parent or other appropriate adult.

The nurse also has an ethical responsibility to prevent illness in patients. Rates of teenage pregnancy vary across the world and are viewed differently depending on the social-cultural contexts in which they occur. It has been estimated that, worldwide, around 13 million children are born each year to women under 20 years of age (Wikipedia 2007). Of these, over 90% of births occur in developing countries, with the highest rate occurring in sub-Saharan Africa where young women tend to marry at a younger age. Teen pregnancies are also a serious issue in the developed world, with the USA having higher rates of births for 15–19 year olds than those of other developed nations (Santelli et al. 2004). In 2000, it was estimated that 333 000 teens under the age of 18 years become pregnant in the USA, with 166 000 of these giving birth (Santelli et al. 2004). Although USA teen pregnancy rates for females aged 15–19 years have declined by 22% over the past decade (from 62.1 per 1000 in 1991 to 48.7 per 1000 in 2000), teen pregnancy, birth and abortion rates remain a significant issue (Gallup-Black & Weitzman 2004).

It is widely acknowledged that teenage pregnancy and early parenthood can lead to 'poor educational achievement, poor physical and mental health, poverty and social isolation' (WHO 2007). Although early parenthood can be a positive experience for young people, it may also have a number of negative health consequences – both for the mother (e.g. preterm labour, maternal anaemia, chest infections, urinary tract infection (Jolly et al. 2000)) and for her infants (e.g. prematurity, lower than average birth weights, higher mortality rates compared to infants born of older women, loss of health benefits from not being breastfed (Swann et al. 2003)).

Although below the legal age of consent, Bobbie has a right to participate in decision making concerning her care and treatment (Cook & Dickens 2000; Dickens & Cook 2005; Sundby 2006). Failing to diagnose Bobbie's pregnancy puts the health of the teenager (and also her fetus) at risk, which the nurse has a responsibility to prevent. However, carrying out this responsibility may mean not fulfilling other responsibilities to the patient, such as enabling her to make an informed choice and to consent to her care and treatment, and to have information about her kept confidential. Thus the value of preventing illness in this case conflicts with the values of people having sufficient information to make informed choices about their care and treatment, and protecting confidentiality. In order to fulfil the nursing responsibility to prevent illness, the nurse must decide how this responsibility should be balanced against the responsibility to ensure the patient is informed and also has information about her kept confidential.

What is the significance of the conflicts to the parties involved?

It might be argued that even though Bobbie is extremely ill, she needs to be informed about the possibility that she is pregnant and to be given the opportunity to consent to a pregnancy test and to being referred to a social worker. It might be further argued that, even though Bobbie is a legal minor, she has the right to decide whether or not her mother is told about Ms Briganti's 'hunch'. It might also be argued, however, that, given how sick Bobbie is, this is a case requiring 'benevolent paternalism' and that the nurse has a role to play both as advocate (of Bobbie's interests) and surrogate decision maker.

What should be done?

It might seem that the simplest solution is for Ms Briganti to ask Bobbie if she is pregnant and, if Bobbie doesn't know, ask her permission to order a pregnancy test. As Bobbie is so ill, however, she may not be able to give a competent response to Ms Briganti's questioning. It might also seem that Bobbie would be better off if her mother knew about the pregnancy. The young woman might not be isolated in her decision making and would have an 'appropriate adult' as a bona fide surrogate decision maker to monitor her health status and medical treatment, and who could consent on her behalf to a pregnancy test being taken. If the nurse truly believes that Bobbie would be better off if the mother knew, breaking her confidence might be an attractive option. However, this would be a subjective evaluation on the nurse's part and might prove to be wrong. (Bobbie might not, in fact, have a functional relationship with her mother.) Respect for Bobbie as a patient means letting her decide whether or not to tell her mother. Thus, if the nurse values keeping confidentiality in the nurse–patient relationship, then she must remain silent in order to preserve Bobbie's trust.

If the nurse believes (and reasons) that her fundamental ethical responsibility to prevent harmful health risks is important, she might seek Bobbie's permission to discuss the situation with either the mother or one of the hospital's social workers. If the teenager agrees, then the nurse would not be overriding her autonomy in speaking to either the mother or the social worker. This course of action would preserve the nurse–patient relationship and would likely benefit Bobbie as well.

If the teenager does not want the nurse to discuss the situation with the mother or a social worker, then the nurse might try other means to persuade Bobbie to be concerned about the potential health risks to herself if pregnant, and also to her fetus if she decides to continue with the pregnancy. She might carefully explain to the teenager the health risks involved. Knowing this, Bobbie might agree to either her mother or the social worker being told and involved, and seek their support. If she chooses not to do this, at the very least she will be in a better position if and when she recovers to decide what to do if she is pregnant. Regardless of the actions chosen, the nurse's responsibility to prevent illness requires that she spend additional time with this teenager to make sure that she has all the information she needs to protect her health, and that she fully understands the potential risks to her health as well as to the health of her fetus. This responsibility can be fulfilled without violating the rights of Bobbie to make informed choices about her care and treatment, and without breaching confidentiality of the nurse–patient relationship. This, in turn, may provide a foundation for future consultations between nurse and patient where Bobbie's health status is concerned.

Case example 10: Preventing female genital mutilation of an infant

What is the story behind the value conflicts?

Robyn Smith is a Maternal and Child Health Nurse (MCHN) who practises in a multi-discipline community health centre which services a growing local population of immigrants and refugees from Africa, the Middle East, Asia and South America. Among its many activities, the community health centre has been working closely with representatives of its immigrant and refugee patient groups on a variety of health promotion and health education programmes. Over the past 12 months, the centre has been particularly active in working with its ethnic community representatives in promoting an education programme aimed at eradicating the harmful traditional practice of female genital mutilation (FGM) or 'female circumcision'. As part of its educational programme and campaign against female genital mutilation, the centre has made it clear that the involuntary circumcision of female children is illegal in this country and would be viewed by the local courts as an assault on the child and a violation of the country's child protection laws. The centre has also advised its staff (including the MCHN) that under existing child protection laws, they are required by law to notify local child protection services of any known or suspected cases of female genital mutilation or children who are at risk of such mutilation.

Mrs Oluloro, a newly arrived refugee, has recently given birth to a baby girl and attends the Maternal and Child Health Clinic as part of a Government funded programme for maternal and child health promoting care. During her second visit to the clinic, Mrs Oluloro confides in the nurse that she is being pressured by her local ethnic community to have her daughter infibulated or 'circumcised'. She explains that if her baby daughter does not have the procedure the consequences will be dire: her daughter will be despised, ridiculed and ultimately ostracised by her local ethnic community. Such a situation would be intolerable both for her daughter and for herself. Mrs Oluloro then asks the nurse if she could recommend a local surgeon who could perform the procedure safely explaining that, if she cannot find a local surgeon to do the operation, her daughter will be left to the mercy of a 'traditional cutter' who had performed the procedure many times in her country of origin. Mrs Oluloro, a well-educated woman, further explains that, although she does not agree with this old traditional practice, she has little choice but to comply in order to avoid the terrible stigma that would befall her daughter, herself and indeed her whole family if the procedure is not carried out. Her baby daughter is three weeks old. How should the nurse respond to this situation?

What is the significance of the values involved?

According to the World Health Organization (WHO), 100 to 140 million girls and women have been genitally mutilated in more than 45 countries and an additional two million girls are at risk annually (Affara 2000, 2002; Reyners 2004; WHO 2000). Of those who have undergone FGM, or who are at risk of FGM, most live in 28 African countries; others live in Asia and the Middle East and are also being increasingly found in the immigrant and refugee populations of Europe, Australia, Canada and the USA (Reyners 2004; WHO 2000). Cutting is traditionally done by 'traditional birth attendants' (e.g. mothers, grandmothers and family friends) or midwives (UNICEF 2007). The tools that are used are often crude and unclean, and the procedure itself is often done without anaesthetic. For Amnesty International, female genital mutilation is 'a human rights issue of huge and compelling proportions'.

FGM is a cultural practice that has been justified on internal cultural grounds that include 'appeals to custom, religion, family honour, cleanliness, aesthetics, initiation, assurance of virginity, promotion of social and political cohesion, enhancement of fertility, improvement in male sexual pleasure, and prevention of female promiscuity' (Sherwin 1992, p. 62; see also Affara 2002; Baron & Denmark 2006; Morris 2006; Reyners 2004). Contrary to popular belief the practice is not supported by any formal doctrine of religion (Braddy & Files 2007). Rather its primary support comes from powerful male religious leaders who have a vested interest in maintaining the subordination of women as well as their own positions of power and control (James 1994).

Today many internal sub-cultural groups of the cultures believed to support FGM are actively working for the eradication of the practice (Johnstone 2004, p. 81; Morris 2006). In the support of the work of these groups, many countries (including some Islamic countries) have outlawed or are working to outlaw the practice. In Sudan, a country commonly associated with infibulation, the practice of FGM has been illegal since 1946, although it still occurs there (West 1994). Moves to eradicate FGM are, therefore, not necessarily a case of western cultural imperialism; rather it is an example of the possibility of achieving a global consensus and action on an important public health and human rights issue and, in doing so, collectively working toward protecting and promoting the moral interests of human beings at risk of harm across the world (Affara 2000, 2002; Baron & Denmark 2006; Hopkins 1999).

The supposed benefits of FGM are highly questionable. There is ample evidence that the practice of FGM fails to achieve a large number of the outcomes desired: the promotion of family honour, cleanliness, aesthetics, assurance of virginity, promotion of social and political cohesion, enhancement of fertility, and the prevention of female promiscuity (Baron & Denmark 2006; Braddy & Files 2007; Johnstone 2004; Morison et al. 2001; Morris 2006; Reyners 2004). On the contrary; the procedure can result in pain, shock, haemorrhage, infection (including an increased risk of contracting HIV/AIDS, hepatitis and tetanus), septicaemia, and gangrene (Baron & Denmark 2006; Ehiemere 1998). FGM also contributes to 'difficulty urinating and menstruating, malformation and scarring of the genitalia, physical and psychological trauma with sexual intercourse, sterility and infant mortality' (James 1994, pp. 8–9; see also Baron & Denmark 2006; Morison et al. 2001; Reyners 2004). It is also known that the procedure does not 'assure virginity' or prevent 'female promiscuity' (Johnstone 2004, p. 81).

What is the significance of the conflicts to the parties involved?

Mrs Oluloro is justified in her concerns about the intolerable social consequences to her daughter, herself and her family if she does not permit the procedure to be carried out. To be ostracised from her ethnic community so soon after arriving in her new country would be devastating and would make adaptation to the new and unfamiliar cultural context she now lives in very difficult. She needs the support that her ethnic community can provide to help her adapt to her new country; without this support, she will not survive.

FGM is, however, illegal in her new country of residence, constitutes a gross violation of human rights and carries a significant and unacceptable risk of causing her daughter a range of physical and psychological harms, some of which will be irreversible. Furthermore, there are members of her own ethnic community who are working actively to try to eradicate the practice. Robyn Smith, the attending nurse, meanwhile, is obliged by law to report the matter to local child protection services. However, Ms Smith is also expected to uphold the agreed ethical standards of the profession which, among other things, requires her to: respect the cultural beliefs and practices of the patients for whom she cares, and to keep information confidential that she has learned in the context of the nurse–patient relationship.

What should be done?

Should Ms Smith simply report the matter to child protection services, as required by law? Or should Ms Smith give Mrs Oluloro the name of a surgeon whom she knows will perform the procedure without risk of the child protection services or other legal authorities finding out? Or should Ms Smith use the opportunity to try to 'educate' Mrs Oluloro to reject the pressure she is being subjected to, to have her daughter 'circumcised'? Would taking this approach, however, be tantamount to cultural imperialism and Ms Smith imposing her own values onto the patient?

This case provides a good example of how nurses need to be well informed about the complexities of human life and the cultural values and beliefs that underpin them. The case also demonstrates how ethical standards governing nursing practice need to be applied in a culturally informed, critically reflective and discretionary manner.

Most nursing codes of ethics and standards of ethical professional conduct (including the ICN *Code of Ethics for Nurses* (2006b)) require nurses to respect the cultural beliefs and practices of their patients, to maintain confidentiality and to take appropriate action to protect the well-being of patients deemed to be at risk of suffering otherwise avoidable harm. Respecting the cultural beliefs and practices of different cultural groups does not mean, however, that the nurse must be totally receptive or subservient to those practices and beliefs – especially when these practices can be shown to be harmful. FGM has been shown to be harmful and morally unacceptable on grounds internal to the cultures which practise it (Baron & Denmark 2006; Braddy & Files 2007; James 1994; Johnstone 2004), as well as by appeal to other standards external to the culture. This convergence of moral opinion makes the rejection and eradication of the practice not only justified, but imperative. As the ICN Position Statement *Elimination of Female Genital Mutilation* (2004) states, 'nurses can act individually, together, and with other organisations to discourage, prevent and eventually eliminate FGM' (p. 1).

It is generally accepted that confidentiality should be maintained in any professional–client relationship, and the nurse–patient relationship is not an exception to this moral rule. The demand to maintain confidentiality, however, is not absolute and may be overridden by other, stronger moral considerations (Johnstone 2004). Nevertheless, any decision by a nurse to breach a confidence must be based on a critical examination of the information and situation at hand, and an evaluation of the expected and desirable moral outcomes that will be achieved by the disclosure of information which has been gained in a confidential professional–client/nurse–patient relationship.

In this case, the interests of Mrs Oluloro's three-week-old baby girl are paramount. In accordance with the nurse's responsibilities to prevent harm and to be an advocate, the significant harm the infant is at risk of suffering ought to be prevented. Complicating this assessment, however, are the long-term social harms the child could suffer by not having the procedure. When considered in the broader context of the local ethnic community's campaign to have FGM eradicated, Mrs Oluloro's fears in this regard may not be as well founded as she thought. Ms Smith must therefore carefully evaluate the harms that both Mrs Oluloro and her baby are at risk of suffering and how best to avert these. This evaluation can best be achieved by a considered, sensitive and well-informed exploration of the issues with Mrs Oluloro who has 'insider' knowledge of the culture which could assist Ms Smith in deciding what to do.

Under law, Ms Smith is required to report the case to child protection services; failure to do so could result in her being penalised. However, her actions could also risk alienating Mrs Oluloro who is dependent on her for much-needed maternal and child healthcare services. In order to meet both her legal and moral responsibilities, Ms Smith needs to communicate fully with Mrs Oluloro (who has already indicated that she does not agree with the practice) and to advise her that, as a nurse, she (Ms Smith) is obliged under law to notify child protection services and that because of this mandated requirement, she cannot keep in confidence the information she has been given. Ms Smith also needs to explain to Mrs Oluloro the processes of making a notification to child protection services, what will happen and explore ways in which the possible harmful impact of this intervention could be minimised and the safety and well-being of her child maximised.

Ms Smith should also seek Mrs Oluloro's consent to locate appropriate support from other women in her ethnic community as well as from mainstream services. By working with Mrs Oluloro, rather than against her, Ms Smith may also contribute to the broader social and ethnic community's educational programmes aimed at eradicating the practice and to secure the promotion and protection of both Mrs Oluloro and her infant daughter's significant moral interests (Affara 2000, 2002; Baron & Denmark 2006; Morris 2006; Reyners 2004).

By following these processes Ms Smith might discover that Mrs Oluloro is, in fact, relieved that something can be done and actually wants the nurse to intervene in order to prevent her baby daughter from being mutilated. With regard to Mrs Oluloro's request for the name of a surgeon who could perform the procedure, it is evident, based on the consideration just discussed, that Ms Smith is under no obligation to provide this requested information. Instead, her overriding obligation is to refer Mrs Oluloro to health professionals and other social service providers who can assist her and provide the support she needs in order to navigate her way out of the cultural prison in which she has found herself.

Exercise:

Case example 11: Putting money where it will prevent the most illness[2]

Rachel T is proposing a community-based illness-prevention programme to the nurse district manager of their clinic. The programme will be designed for unmarried teenagers who have had one child out of wedlock. The goal is to reduce the risk of a repeat pregnancy and the potential for low-birth-weight infants by providing contraceptive services and friendly support. It also aims to prevent childhood illnesses among the teenagers' children by providing frequent health examinations for the child, child immunisations, child care services and child development teaching. The programme will be of moderate cost, require two nurses and will serve approximately 60 teenagers a year.

Yakov C is also proposing an illness-prevention programme for the clinic. His programme will be designed for elderly people living in single-resident units. The goal is to reduce the number of admissions to local emergency rooms through nurse monitoring of medication usage, home safety check-ups, routine health check-ups, a telephone service for home-bound patients and a low cost, one-meal-a-day service. The cost of the programme will be moderately high and require one full-time nurse and two nursing assistants. It will serve approximately 100 elderly citizens.

The nurse district manager must use her financial resources where it will serve the greatest number of citizens in the community and have the greatest impact on short-term illness-prevention for political reasons. She would like to support both programmes but does not have the financial resources to do so. How can she ethically justify choosing one programme and not the other?

Discussion questions

What is the story behind the value conflicts?

(1) What is the ethical problem faced by the district manager in this case example?

(2) What are the values involved from Rachel T's view? From Yakov C's view? From the nurse district manager's view?

What is the significance of the values involved?

(3) What are the meanings of these values to each person involved? Which values seem to be in conflict?

(4) Are there any legal or professional practice questions involved in this case example?

What is the significance of the conflicts to the parties involved?

(5) How might the health of individuals served by the clinic be affected by each illness-prevention programme?

(6) What kind of illness-prevention policies might be represented by each programme, if adopted and funded?

What should be done?

(7) What are the probable outcomes if the district manager decides to initiate the programme serving unmarried teenage mothers? The programme serving the elderly living alone?

(8) What are the criteria that the district manager should use to select a programme for funding? Why? Are the criteria ethical? Why or why not?

(9) Which programme should she initiate? Why?

(10) Should she attempt to initiate both programmes on a reduced scale? Why or why not?

Planning community health programmes presents an interesting dilemma for the clinic's district manager. Because she is removed from a direct relationship with individual patients who might participate in the proposed programmes, she can make a decision that balances individual good with collective good. She can do this because there is no danger of harming any pre-existing relationship with any of the potential patients. Her judgment will reflect her knowledge of the agency's criteria and priorities for disbursement of monies and her experience with previous illness-prevention programmes initiated by the nursing staff. It may create many value conflicts for her nursing staff and she will need to be prepared to assist the staff nurses to understand and resolve these conflicts.

As district manager, she will probably want to see a needs assessment for each planned programme, the results of a projection study for each programme in terms of health goods promoted and illness prevented, and a cost-effectiveness analysis for each programme. She will probably make a decision based on serving the greatest need at the least cost and will need to justify this decision ethically. This may be difficult to do because it is not certain which programme will contribute the most to these desirable outcomes or if some combination of both programmes will be best.

Summary

The responsibility to prevent illness can create value conflicts for the practising nurse. The conflicts may involve values related to patient self-determination and patient well-being and may often involve professional values such as privacy, confidentiality and keeping promises to patients. Nurses in administrative and managerial positions may experience value conflicts when they attempt to prevent illness among patient populations through programmes that target or favour one population or age group over another. In these instances, the responsibility to prevent illness will need to be clarified as to whether it applies primarily to individual health, or to the aggregate health of community members.

Notes

1   Adapted from Fry, S.T. & Veatch, R.M. (2006) *Case studies in nursing ethics*, 3rd ed. Boston: Jones & Bartlett, Publishers (pp. 176–177). Used with permission.
2   Adapted from Fry, S.T. & Veatch, R.M. (2006) *Case studies in nursing ethics*, 3rd ed. Boston: Jones & Bartlett, Publishers (pp. 111–112). Used with permission.

References

Affara, F.A. (2000) When tradition maims. *AJN* 100(8), 52–61.
Affara, F.A. (2002) Guest editorial: Female genital mutilation is a human rights issue of concern to all women and men. *International Nursing Review* 49(4), 195–197.
Baron, E.M. & Denmark, F.L. (2006) An exploration of female genital mutilation. *Ann NY Acad Sci* 1087(1), 339–355.
Braddy, C.M. & Files, J.A. (2007) Female genital mutilation: Cultural awareness and clinical considerations. *J of Midwifery & Women's Health* 52(2), 158–163.
Cameron, M.E. (1993) *Living with AIDS*. Newbury Park, CA: Sage Publications.
Committee on Economic, Social and Cultural Rights (CESCR) (2000) *The right to the highest attainable standard of health*. General Comment No. 14. Geneva: Office of the United Nations High Commissioner for Human Rights.
Cook, R. & Dickens, B. (2000) Recognizing adolescents' 'evolving capacities' to exercise choice in reproductive healthcare. *Int J of Gynecol Obstet* 70, 13–21.
Derish, M. & Vanden Heuvel, K. (2000) Mature minors should have the right to refuse life-sustaining medical treatment. *Journal of Law, Medicine and Ethics* 28, 109–24.
Dickens, B. & Cook, R. (2005) Ethical and legal issues in reproductive health: adolescents and consent to treatment. *Int. J. of Gynecol and Obstet* 89, 179–184.

Ehiemere, I.O. (1998) Cultural practices: Issues and problems on health of our communities. *W African J Nurs* 9(2), 95–98.

Foster, C. & Lyall, H. (2005) Current guidelines for the management of UK infants born to HIV-1 infected mothers. *Early Human Development* 81(1), 103–110.

Fry, S.T. & Veatch, R.M. (2006) *Case studies in nursing ethics*, 3rd ed. Boston: Jones & Bartlett Publishers.

Gallup-Black, A. & Weitzman, B. (2004) Teen pregnancy and urban youth: competing truths, complacency, and perceptions of the problem. *Journal of Adolescent Health* 34(5), 366–375.

Grady, D. (1995) *The search for an AIDS vaccine*. Bloomington, IN: Indiana University Press.

Harris, P. & Siplon, P. (2001) International obligation and human health: evolving policy responses to HIV/AIDS. *Ethics & International Affairs* 15(2), 29–52.

Hopkins, S. (1999) A discussion of the legal aspects of female genital mutilation. *J Adv. Nurs* 30(4), 926–933.

Hunt, M. (2004) AIDS: Globalization and its discontents. *Zygon* 39(2), 465–480.

International Council of Nurses (ICN) (2000) *Position statement: Health information: protecting patients' rights*. Geneva, Switzerland: ICN.

International Council of Nurses (ICN) (2001) *Position statement: Acquired immunodeficiency syndrome (AIDS)*. Geneva, Switzerland: ICN.

International Council of Nurses (ICN) (2004) *Position statement: Elimination of female genital mutilation*. Geneva, Switzerland: ICN.

International Council of Nurses (ICN) (2006a) *Position statement: Nurses and human rights*. Geneva, Switzerland: ICN.

International Council of Nurses (ICN) (2006b) *Code of ethics for nurses*. Geneva, Switzerland: ICN.

James, S. (1994) Reconciling international human rights and cultural relativism: the case of female circumcision. *Bioethics* 8(1), 1–26.

Johnstone, M.J. (2004) *Bioethics: A nursing perspective*, 4th ed. Sydney: Elsevier Science/Churchill Livingstone.

Jolly, M., Sebire, N., Harris, J., Robinson, S. & Regan, L. (2000) Obstetric risk of pregnancy in women less than 18 years old. *Obstetrics & Gynecology* 96(6), 962–966.

Kourtis, A., Bulterys, M., Nesheim, S. & Lee, F. (2001) Understanding the timing of HIV transmission from mother to infant. *JAMA* 285(6), 709–712.

Kourtis, A., Lee, F., Abrams, E., Jamieson, D. & Bulterys, M. (2006) Mother-to-child transmission of HIV-1: timing and implications for prevention. *Lancet Infect Dis* 6(11), 726–732.

Kuhn, L., Steketee, R., Weedon, J., Abrams, E., Lambert, G., Bamji, M., Schoenbaum, E., Farley, J., Nesheim, S., Palumbo, P., Simonds, R. & Thea, D. (1999) Distinct risk factors for intrauterine and intrapartum human immunodeficiency virus transmission and consequences for disease progression in infected children. Perinatal AIDS Collaboration Transmission Study. *J Infect Dis* 179(1), 52–58.

Lehrer, J., Pantell, R., Tebb, K. & Shafer, M. (2007) Forgone health care among US adolescents: association between risk characteristics and confidentiality concern. *Journal of Adolescent Health* 40, 218–226.

Morison, L., Scherf, C., Ekpo, G., Paine, K., West, B., Coleman, R. & Walraven, G. (2001) The long-term reproductive health consequences of female genital cutting in rural Gambia: a community-based survey. *Tropical Medicine & International Health* 6(8), 643–653.

Morris, K. (2006) Feature issues on female genital mutilation/cutting – progress and parallels. *The Lancet* 368, 564–566.

Ostergren, M. & Malyuta, R. (2006) Elimination of HIV infection in infants in Europe – challenges and demand for response. *Seminars in Fetal & Neonatal Medicine* 11(1), 54–57.

Petropoulou, H., Stratigos, A. & Katsambas, A. (2006) Human immunodeficiency virus infection and pregnancy. *Clinics in Dermatology* 24(6), 536–542.

Poku, N. (2006) HIV/AIDS financing: a case for improving the quality and quantity of aid. *International Affairs* 82(2), 345–358.

Reyners, M. (2004) Health consequences of female genital mutilation. *Reviews in Gynaecological Practice* 4(4), 242–251.

Rosenberg, T. (January 28, 2001) The world's AIDS crisis is solvable: Look at Brazil. *New York Times Magazine*, pp. 26–31, 52, 58, 62–63.

Sanci, L., Sawyer, S., Kang, M., Haller, D. & Patton, G. (2005) Confidential health care for adolescents: reconciling clinical evidence with family values. *Medical Journal of Australia* 183(8), 410–414.

Santelli, J., Abma, J., Ventura, S. et al. (2004) Can changes in sexual behaviours among high school students explain the decline in teen pregnancy rates in the 1990s? *Journal of Adolescent Health* 35(2), 80–90.

Sherwin, S. (1992) *No longer patient: Feminist ethics & health care.* Philadelphia: Temple University Press.

Sundby, J. (2006) Young people's sexual and reproductive health rights. *Best Practice & Research Clinical Obstetrics & Gynaecology* 20(3), 355–368.

Swann, C., Bowe, K., McCormick, G. & Kosmin, M. (2003) *Teenage pregnancy and parenthood: A review of reviews.* Wetherby, Yorkshire: NHS Health Development Agency.

UNAIDS/WHO (2006) *Dec06: AIDS epidemic update.* Joint United Nations Programme on HIV/AIDS (UNAIDS) and World Health Organisation [available at: http://www.unaids.org/en/HIV_data/epi2006/ – accessed 26 November 2007].

UNICEF (2007) *Child protection from violence, exploitation and abuse: Female genital mutilation* [available at: http://www.unicef.org/proection/index_genitalmutilation.html?q=printme – accessed 3 August 2007].

West, R. (1994) Education better than bans, say African women. *The Age* (Melbourne) 17 February, p. 6.

Wikipedia (2007) Teenage pregnancy. Wikipedia®. Available at: http://en.wikipedia.org (accessed 8 March 2007).

World Health Organization (WHO) (2000) *Female genital mutilation.* Fact sheet No. 241. Geneva: WHO.

World Health Organization (WHO) (2002) *25 questions & answers on health & human rights.* Geneva: WHO.

World Health Organization (WHO) (2006a) *Taking stock: health worker shortages and the response to AIDS.* Geneva: WHO.

World Health Organization (WHO) (2006b) *Global AIDS epidemic continues to grow.* News release 21 November 2006. Geneva: WHO.

World Health Organization (WHO) (2007) *What are the most effective strategies for reducing the rate of teenage pregnancies?* Geneva: WHO.

Zanetti, A., Tanzi, E. & Semprini, A. (2006) Hepatitis C in pregnancy and mother-to-infant transmission of HCV. *Perspectives in Medical Virology* 13, 153–171.

Chapter 8
Restoring health

R ... f nursing practice through-
ou ... personnel enter and exit
th ... uchstone for patient and
fa ... , therefore, play key roles
in ... cepts of advocacy, caring,
cc ... le for establishing a milieu
w ... ral practices and customs
ca

a ... various obligations associ-
e ... r the nurse, or the nurse's
f ... y's values and beliefs. The
ta ... nvolved in restoring men-
... d religious belief systems.

... h a potential

... in a country experiencing
... ealthcare effort. Although she
anticipated many cultural, religious and social differences in the way that healthcare is provided in this country, she finds it difficult to accept the subservient role
of women in this society. She is particularly concerned about Mrs Ahmed, a young
mother with three small daughters who recently visited the health clinic for treatment of severe diarrhoea in her youngest child.

Mrs Ahmed was born and educated in a western country. After completing
her studies, she married Mr Ahmed, a Muslim, and returned with him to his country. A few months later, civil war broke out in their country and Mrs Ahmed lost
all contact with her western friends and relatives.

When Ms Schmidt first met Mrs Ahmed, she was troubled by the young mother's frail, withdrawn appearance. After several visits, Ms Schmidt begins to suspect that the intelligent young woman is suffering from a mental illness (severe depression). Being confined at home with the children, not entirely accepted by her husband's family, and limited (according to her husband's cultural and religious beliefs) in her opportunity to socialise with others outside the family, all contribute to her feelings of extreme loneliness and fear. In her husband's family, Mrs Ahmed must maintain a subservient role in keeping with the society's beliefs and teach her own daughters to do the same. Mrs Ahmed confides that she fears that she will never again see her native country or her parents and siblings. She is also afraid that her children will never know any customs other than those of their father's family and country. Because Mrs Ahmed is not accepted by the husband's family, Ms Schmidt is uncertain whether anyone in the family recognises that the young woman is suffering from a mental illness. How does the nurse carry out her ethical responsibility to restore health where this patient is concerned?

What is the significance of the values involved?

Providing healthcare in a foreign country can prove a rigorous test of a nurse's ethics and personal values and beliefs. A nurse is usually obligated to treat illness and restore health in any patient under her care. When carrying out this responsibility means confronting deeply held cultural, religious and social values and beliefs, the obligation is not as clear. When the restoration of health means treatment for mental illness, the obligation becomes even less clear.

How should Ms Schmidt, a nurse with entirely different cultural and religious-based value systems, discuss Mrs Ahmed's mental health problems with the patient's husband and his family members? Should she reveal her concerns about the roles that the cultural and religious values and cultural belief systems of Mr Ahmed and his family are playing in the wife's illness?

`The values held by the parties in this situation vary widely. Mrs Ahmed, Mr Ahmed, his family members and Ms Schmidt all have very different belief systems and values, each of which holds important meanings for each individual. Ms Schmidt's nursing practice will certainly be influenced by the Ahmed family's values. On the other hand, enforcing her values on Mrs Ahmed could have an adverse effect on the patient and her willingness to work closely with the nurse in restoring her mental health (Andary et al. 2003; Campinha-Bacote 2002; Donnelly 2000; Holland & Hogg 2001; Mahoney & Engebretson 2000).

What is the significance of the conflicts to the parties involved?

If Mrs Ahmed were suffering from a noticeable physical ailment, the nurse would not hesitate to implement a culturally relevant plan of care to restore the woman's physical health. However, suffering from a mental illness while living in a social-cultural context in which mental illness is highly stigmatised, and where women (and women's health) are disadvantaged, can be very difficult (Jecker, Carrese & Pearlman 1995; St Hill et al. 2003; Solheim 2005). There is no simple way to restore Mrs Ahmed's mental health without creating value conflict for the nurse and for Mrs Ahmed. A culturally informed, appropriate and responsive approach to nursing care delivery can be helpful in these types of situations because they take into consideration the impact and effects that the cultural values and beliefs of *both* health service provider and patient can have on healthcare practices and patient health outcomes (Andary et al. 2003; Holland & Hogg 2001; Johnstone & Kanitsaki 2006; Papadopoulos 2006; Smedley et al. 2003). It is hoped that such approaches can be used in this situation to help restore Mrs Ahmed's mental health with the least possible value conflict.

What should be done?

Ms Schmidt has an obligation to be truthful with the husband and should faithfully attempt to enlist the husband's help in caring for Mrs Ahmed (Moazam 2000). If there are culturally relevant measures that can be employed to help treat his wife's mental health problems, the husband and/or his family could be an important resource in discovering what these measures might be. Thus, the first step in carrying out the ethical obligation to restore health may be for the nurse to clearly communicate her observations to the patient's husband and family (Andary et al. 2003; Jubb & Shanley 2002; Muñoz & Luckman 2005).

Understanding and respect for the culture of the Ahmeds are also important to the success of any plan that might be initiated to prevent further deterioration of Mrs Ahmed's mental health (ICN 2002). The family unit is often the most important social organisation in cultural groups and may take on a pivotal role in providing healthcare to and restoring health in a loved one (Chang 2001; Dudley & Carr 2004; Jubb & Shanley 2002; Meyers et al. 2004). If possible, the family's status and importance in the cultural group should be viewed by the nurse as part of the solution to an ethical and healthcare issue, rather than part of the problem (Åstedt-Kurki et al. 2001; Johnstone 2004; Kuczewski 1996). The nurse's obligation to restore health must be carried out with respect for the cultural, religious and social values of the patient and his or her family unit (Holland & Hogg 2001; Kanitsaki 1993; Leininger & McFarland 2006; Purnell & Paulanka 2003).

Last, Ms Schmidt should recommend out-patient psychiatric follow-up to keep Mrs Ahmed in touch with the healthcare system outside of the family group. This contact would enhance her recovery and support her own values and beliefs that should not be denied. Judgments about mental illness often reflect one's own values and beliefs about what constitutes mental health within one's own cultural group. In the final analysis, Mrs Ahmed's successful restoration to full mental health will depend, in several respects, on how mental health is perceived and what meanings are given to it by both her husband and his family, as well as the level of congruency between their cultural values, beliefs and practices in regard to mental health, and those of the healthcare team. By being recommended out-patient psychiatric follow-up, Mrs Ahmed will be helped to accommodate her own values and beliefs with those of her husband and his family without denying the relevance and importance of any of them.

The ethical obligation to restore health provides support for many innovative healthcare services throughout the world. In fact, the increasing use of technology in healthcare has made the restoration of health a big business in many countries, dramatically changing nursing practice in some areas. Heart valves, hips joints and knee parts can be replaced by synthetic materials, enabling the patient to resume a previous or even improved lifestyle. Kidney stones can be removed without major surgical intervention and chronic diseases such as arthritis can be ameliorated by powerful chemical agents. However, one of the most successful conventional means of treating both fatal and nonfatal diseases and restoring individual health is solid organ transplantation (WHO 2003).

Although ethically controversial in some contexts, successful organ transplantation can improve a person's quality of life and increase their lifespan; it even promises to decrease the costs associated with maintenance of many chronic diseases such as kidney or liver diseases (Emiroglu et al. 2005; Mutimer 2007; Port et al. 2004; Rizvi & Naqvi 2000; Sanchez-Bueno et al. 2005; WHO 2003). Nurses are often viewed as having a key role to play in the procurement and transplantation of organs that includes identifying potential organ donors, and caring for donors, organ recipients and their families (Boey 2002; Collins 2005; Conesa et al. 2005; DeVeaux 2006; Frid et al. 1998; Kim et al. 2006). In fulfilling these roles, however, ethical questions often arise. The following case example demonstrates some of these questions.

Case example 13: Are some patients more worthy than others?

What is the story behind the value conflicts?

Olga Nordstrom cares for three patients who are awaiting donated kidneys from cadavers. Mrs A, a 45-year-old housewife with three pre-adolescent children, has been on the transplant waiting list the longest – two years. Her condition is progressively deteriorating from many complications. Mr B, a 63-year-old retired businessman and a widower, has been on the waiting list for three months. He is very seriously ill due to kidney failure following a recent suicide attempt. He has suffered periodic bouts of severe depression since his wife died in a car accident four years previously. Mr C, a 39-year-old unemployed labourer with a history of drug and alcohol abuse, has been on the waiting list for a cadaver kidney for 14 months. He has no living children and lives with an older sister who provides him with supportive care.

Within a week, both Mr B and Mr C receive donor kidneys and are successfully transplanted. Mrs A's condition continues to deteriorate and she dies before another kidney becomes available. Ms Nordstrom believes that inequities must exist in the organ donation system because Mrs A was on the list the longest and had a positive role to play in the lives of her children. Over time, she finds it hard to provide close support to waiting patients and their families because she knows that some patients will not receive an organ and will die as a result. How should Mrs Nordstrom resolve the nagging questions she has about the fairness of the organ transplant system and her ethical obligations to patients under her care?

What is the significance of the values involved?

Organ donation rates vary across the world, ranging from 20.7 donors per million in North America and 17.2 donors per million in Europe, to just 2.06 donors per million in Africa and 1.1 per million in Asia (PAHO–WHO 2005). In all instances, organ donation rates are lower than treatment incidence rates (PAHO–WHO 2005). In recent years, organ donation rates have fallen in some developed nations (e.g. UK, USA) despite these nations having considerable healthcare resources available (Abadie & Gay 2006; PAHO–WHO 2005; Port et al. 2004). Thus, although organ transplantation programmes save and prolong thousands of lives each year, organ supply is generally insufficient to meet demand and reduce the number of people on a waiting list for a transplant (PAHO–WHO 2003).

Caring for patients who are awaiting transplantation can be a painful as well as rewarding experience for all involved. When a patient receives an organ and it is successfully transplanted, his or her health is restored. Caring for such a patient is generally a positive experience for the nurse. However, when a patient's condition declines while waiting to be transplanted, caring for the patient becomes emotionally painful because his or her death is certain. In these situations, nurses may question the fairness and equity of cadaver organ distribution. The nurse may even begin to believe that he or she has personally failed the patient. If a cadaver organ is not available for the patient, the patient's health cannot be restored and the nurse has not been able to fulfil an ethical responsibility toward this goal. This may create value conflicts for the nurse and tensions among the health-care team (DeVeaux 2006; Frid et al. 1998; Pearson et al. 2001; Regehr et al. 2004).

When families learn that an organ will not be available in time to save their loved one, the nurse will be expected to respond to family members' questions about the system of organ distribution. In addition, the nurse may need to discuss the feasibility of organ donation by living relatives or by unrelated donors if cadaver organs are unavailable. Finally, the nurse may need to understand how different cultural, religious and ethical values and beliefs influence patient and family attitudes toward cadaver organs and respond to questions concerning why one patient received an organ and another did not (Abadie & Gay 2006; Bagheri 2005; Boey 2002; Mizraji et al. 2007).

What is the significance of the conflicts to the parties involved?

To carry out their ethical responsibility to patients and family members, nurses must first be knowledgeable about the transplantation system used in their country and know how people are admitted to the waiting list for cadaver organs. As a result of the scarcity of available cadaver organs, many patients will never receive a donor organ and will die. Long waiting lists also exist in other countries where the use of limited cadaver organs is further complicated by cultural and religious belief systems (Abadie & Gay 2006; Bagheri 2005; Boey 2002; Mizraji et al. 2007; Yeung, Kong & Lee 2000).

Recognising that organ transplantation is an altruistic practice involving the gift of a body organ from one person to another person who needs the organ in order to live, the Fortieth World Health Assembly adopted a draft set of principles to guide human organ transplantation (WHO 1991) (Figure 8.1). The purpose of the principles (still in operation today) is 'to provide an orderly, ethical and acceptable framework for regulating the acquisition and transplantation of human organs for therapeutic purposes' (WHO 1991, p. 7). They explicitly prohibit commercial transactions with donated organs, coercion and/or improper inducement to minors and other vulnerable persons to donate their organs.

What should be done?

Understanding these principles is necessary if the nurse is to carry out his or her ethical responsibility adequately to patients awaiting organ transplantation and to those considering donation of their own, or a family member's, organs. Nurses contribute significantly to restoration of health in the community when they educate community members about the issues associated with organ donation and can explain the organ donation and tracking system of their country. Their close contact with families and individual patients often makes nurses the initial communicator to potential organ donors. In caring for patients like Mrs A, Mr B and

Guiding principle 1:
Organs may be removed from the bodies of deceased persons for the purpose of transplantation if:
- Any consents required by law are obtained; and
- There is no reason to believe that the deceased person objected to such removal, in the absence of any formal consent given during the person's lifetime.

Guiding principle 2:
Physicians determining that the death of a potential donor has occurred should not be directly involved in organ removal from the donor and subsequent transplantation procedures, or be responsible for the care of potential recipients of such organs.

Guiding principle 3:
Organs for transplantation should be removed preferably from the bodies of deceased persons. However, adult living persons may donate organs, but in general such donors should be genetically related to the recipients. Exceptions may be made in the case of transplantation of bone marrow and other acceptable regenerative tissues.
  An organ may be removed from the body of an adult living donor for the purpose of transplantation if the donor gives free consent. The donor should be free of any undue influence and pressure and sufficiently informed to be able to understand and weigh the risks, benefits and consequences of consent.

Guiding principle 4:
No organ should be removed from the body of a living minor for the purpose of transplantation. Exceptions may be made under national law in the case of regenerative tissues.

Guiding principle 5:
The human body and its parts cannot be the subject of commercial transactions. Accordingly, giving or receiving payment (including any other compensation or reward) for organs should be prohibited.

Guiding principle 6:
Advertising the need for or availability of organs, with a view to offering or seeking payment, should be prohibited.

Guiding principle 7:
It should be prohibited for physicians and other health professionals to engage in organ transplantation procedures if they have reason to believe that the organs concerned have been the subject of commercial transactions.

Guiding principle 8:
It should be prohibited for any person or facility involved in organ transplantation procedures to receive any payment that exceeds a justifiable fee for the services rendered.

Guiding principle 9:
In the light of the principles of distributive justice and equity, donated organs should be made available to patients on the basis of medical need and not on the basis of financial or other considerations.

Figure 8.1   Guiding principles on human organ transplantation (World Health Organization 1991).

Mr C, the nurse has an opportunity to contribute significantly to the information needs of the organ transplant recipient and donors. Although some patients may not receive an organ transplant, this may reflect cultural practices rather than inequities related to the healthcare system and, especially, the care provided by the nurse. The responsibility to restore health is a strong ethical responsibility of the nurse. However, there will be times when a patient's health cannot be restored and the nurse then must shift his or her attention to the ethical responsibility to alleviate suffering (Fry & Veatch 2006; Kahn & Steeves 1986).

Increased understanding of the ethical principles guiding organ transplantation and the nature of ethical responsibility to the patient will certainly help nurses like Mrs Nordstrom who provide care for transplant recipients, and who are important sources of information for family members and the community where organ donation is concerned. Understanding the ethical issues associated with organ donation is also important to the capacity of nurses to provide ethical care.

Exercise:

Case example 14: The duty to restore health in those who demonstrate against the organisation

T Lagowski is a clinic nurse at a large public university. Recent changes in the country's government and economic hardship have created many tensions in her country. One day, a number of university students stage a demonstration against governmental reforms. The demonstration becomes a riot and university property is damaged. Several students are killed and many others are wounded by the police or are injured in trying to avoid the demonstrators. Several of the students (one of them is the main leader of the demonstration) seek first aid treatment for their injuries at the university health clinic.

The following day, university officials ask to see Mrs Lagowski's clinic records so they can see the names of the students she treated. She knows that the police are continuing to look for the leaders of the demonstration. She refuses, telling the officials that divulging the names of the students treated will constitute a breach of their rights to confidentiality. She also views intervention by university officials as interfering with her ethical obligation to restore health to students who need nursing care. A university official tells her she must give him this information because she is a paid employee of the state and her first obligation is to the public organisation, not to individual students. She practises nursing at the will of the country. Furthermore, he considers the students to be troublemakers who should be punished. Mrs Lagowski disagrees with this position but she is not sure she can prevent the officials from confiscating her records. What should she do? Will her job (and possibly even her personal safety and life) be in jeopardy if she refuses to hand over the names of the students? Does she have an obligation to yield to university pressure in order to stay in her position? In other words, is it better to continue to provide some care to the students than none at all?

Discussion questions

What is the story behind the value conflicts?

    (1) How would Ms Lagowski define the ethical conflict(s) in this story? How would the university officials define the ethical conflict(s) from their perspective? How would the university students whom Ms Lagowski treated define the ethical conflict(s)?

    (2) What are the values involved in each perspective of the ethical conflict(s)?

What is the significance of the values involved?

    (3) What are the meanings of the values from each perspective on the ethical conflict(s)? .

    (4) If Ms Lagowski tells the university officials the names of the students that she treated, are there any legal or professional questions about this action? Why or why not?

    (5) Which values constitute the greatest ethical conflict in this situation?

What is the significance of the conflicts to the parties involved?

    (6) How significant are the value conflicts to Ms Lagowski herself? To the university students? To the university officials?

    (7) If Mrs Lagowski is pressured to tell the names of the students she treated, how might the value conflicts influence nursing practice in a university health centre setting?

    (8) How might this influence the use of the health clinic by the university students?

    (9) What kind of policies could prevent these types of value conflicts from occurring in the future? Is policy desirable to prevent these value conflicts from occurring? Why or why not?

What should be done?

    (10) How should the value conflicts be resolved?

    (11) What are the possible outcomes of their resolution?

    (12) Which moral judgments or actions should Ms Lagowski follow in this situation? Why?

Summary

The ethical responsibility to restore health may give rise to value conflicts in nursing care. Patients' cultural and religious values and beliefs may impinge on the nurse's values and beliefs, and vice versa. When delivering nursing care in a foreign country or in a cultural environment with which the nurse is not familiar, nurses need to work within the cultural values and belief system of that country or environment in order to fulfil their ethical responsibilities as a nurse. When technological developments and innovative treatments are unavailable, or perhaps even prohibited for political and/or social-cultural reasons, nurses may need to reinterpret what the ethical responsibility to restore health means within that system. Each patient's health cannot always be restored and the nurse is not morally responsible for all aspects of an individual's health status. Nurses are responsible, however, to use whatever reasonable means are available to them to promote the health of others so they can achieve the highest attainable standard of health available to them.

References

Abadie, A. & Gay, S. (2006) The impact of presumed consent legislation on cadaveric organ donation: a cross-country study. *Journal of Health Economics* 25(4), 599–620.

Andary, L., Stolk, Y. & Klimidis, S. (2003) *Assessing mental health across cultures*. Bowen Hills, Qld: Australian Academic Press.

Åstedt-Kurki, P., Paavilainen, E., Tammentie, T. & Paunoen-Ilmonen, M. (2001) Interactions between family members and health care providers in an acute care setting in Finland. *Journal of Family Nursing* 7(4), 371–390.

Bagheri, A. (2005) Organ transplantation laws in Asian countries: a comparative study. *Transplantation Proceedings* 37, 4159–4162.

Boey, K. (2002) A cross-validation study of nurses' attitudes and commitment to organ donation in Hong Kong. *International Journal of Nursing Studies* 39, 95–104.

Campinha-Bacote, J. (2002) Cultural competence in psychiatric nursing: have you 'asked' the right questions? *Journal of the American Psychiatric Nurses Association* 8(6), 183–187.

Chang, L. (2001) Family at the bedside: strength of the Chinese family or weakness of hospital care? *Current Sociology* 49(3), 155–173.

Collins, T. (2005) Organ and tissue donation: a survey of nurse's knowledge and educational needs in an adult ITU. *Intensive and Critical Care Nursing* 21, 226–233.

Conesa, C., Ríos, A., Ramírez, P., Sánchez, J., Sánchez, M., Rodríguez, M., Martínez, L., Ramos, F. & Parrilla, P. (2005) Attitude of primary care nurses toward living kidney donation. *Transplantation Proceedings* 37(9), 3626–3630.

DeVeaux, T. (2006) Non-heart-beating organ donation: issues and ethics for the critical care nurse. *Journal of Vascular Nursing* 24(1), 17–21.

Donnelly, P. (2000) Ethics and cross-cultural nursing. *Journal of Transcultural Nursing* 11(2), 119–126.

Dudley, S. & Carr, J. (2004) Vigilance: the experience of parents staying at the bedside of hospitalized children. *Journal of Psychiatric Nursing* 19(4), 267–275.

Emiroglu, R., Moray, G., Sevmis, S., Sözen, M., Bilgin, N. & Haberal, M. (2005) Long term results of pediatric kidney transplantation at one center in Turkey. *Transplantation Proceedings* 37, 2951–2953.

Frid, I., Bergbom-Engberg, & Haljamäe, H. (1998) Brain death in ICUs and associated nursing care challenges concerning patients and families. *Intensive and Critical Care Nursing* 14(1), 21–29.

Fry, S.T. & Veatch, R.M. (2006) *Case studies in nursing ethics*, 3rd ed. Boston: Jones & Bartlett, Publishers.

Holland, K. & Hogg, C. (2001) *Cultural awareness in nursing and health care*. London: Arnold.

International Council of Nurses (ICN) (2002) *Position statement: Mental health.* Geneva, Switzerland: ICN.

Jecker, N.S., Carrese, J.A. & Pearlman, R.A. (1995) Caring for patients in cross-cultural settings. *Hast Ctr Rprt* 25, 6–14.

Johnstone, M. (2004) *Bioethics: A nursing perspective*, 4th ed. Sydney: Elsevier/Churchill Livingstone.

Johnstone, M. & Kanitsaki, O. (2006) Culture, language and patient safety: making the link. *International Journal for Quality in Health Care* 18(5), 383–388.

Jubb, M. & Shanley, E. (2002) Family involvement: the key to opening locked wards and closed minds. *International Journal of Mental Health Nursing* 11, 47–53.

Kahn, D. & Steeves, R. (1986) The experience of suffering: conceptual clarification and theoretical definition. *Journal of Advanced Nursing* 11(6), 623–631.

Kanitsaki, O. (1993) Transcultural human care: Its challenge to and critique of professional nursing care. In D.A. Gaut, *A global agenda for caring* (pp. 19–45). New York: National League for Nursing.

Kim, J., Fisher, M. & Elliott, D. (2006) Undergraduate nursing students' knowledge and attitudes towards organ donation in Korea: implications for education. *Nurse Education Today* 26(6), 465–474.

Kuczewski, M. (1996) Preconceiving the family: the process of consent in medical decisionmaking. *Hast Ctr Rprt* 26(2), 30–37.

Leininger, M. & McFarland, M. (Eds) (2006) *Culture care diversity & universality: A theory*, 2nd ed. Boston: Jones & Bartlett.

Mahoney, J. & Engebretson, J. (2000) The interface of anthropology and nursing guiding culturally competent care in psychiatric nursing. *Archives of Psychiatric Nursing* XIV(4), 183–190.

Meyers, T., Eichhorn, D., Guzzetta, C., Clark, A. & Taliaferro, E. (2004) Family presence during invasive procedures and resuscitation. *Topics in Emergency Medicine* 26(1), 61–73.

Mizraji, R., Alvarez, R., Palacios, C., Fajardo, C., Berrios, F., Morales, E. et al. (2007) Organ donation in Latin America. *Transplantation Proceedings* 39, 333–335.

Moazam, F. (2000) Families, patients, and physicians in medical decision making: a Pakistani perspective. *Hast Ctr Rprt* 30(6), 28–37.

Muñoz, C. & Luckman, J. (2005) *Transcultural communication in nursing*, 2nd ed. Clifton Park, NY: Thomson/Delmar Learning.

Mutimer, D. (2007) Liver transplantation. *Medicine* 35(2), 112–115.

Pan American Health Organization–World Health Organization (PAHO–WHO) (2003) Report by the secretariat, 113 Session, Provisional Agenda Item 3.17, EB113/14, 27 November 2003.

Pan American Health Organization–World Health Organization (PAHO–WHO) (2005) *39th Session of the Subcommittee on Planning and Programming of the Executive Council: Strengthening of National Programs for Organ Donations and Transplants.* Washington DC: PAHO–WHO.

Papadopoulos, I. (2006) *Transcultural health and social care: Development of culturally competent practitioners.* Edinburgh: Elsevier/Churchill Livingstone.

Pearson, A., Roberston-Malt, S., Walsh, K., & Fitzgerald, M. (2001) Intensive care nurses' experiences of caring for brain dead organ donor patients. *Journal of Clinical Nursing* 10(1), 132–139.

Port, F., Dykstra, D., Merion, R. & Wolfe, R. (2004) Organ donation and transplantation trends in the USA, 2003. *American Journal of Transplantation*, 4(Supp. 9), 7–12.

Purnell, L. & Paulanka, B. (2003) *Transcultural health care: A culturally competent approach.* Philadelphia: F.A. Davis.

Regehr, C., Kjerulf, M., Popova, S. & Baker, A. (2004) Trauma and tribulation: the experiences and attitudes of operating room nurses working with organ donors. *Journal of Clinical Nursing* 13(4), 430–437.

Rizvi, S.A.H. & Naqvi, S.A.A. (2000) Our vision on organ donation in developing countries. *Transplantation Proceedings* 32, 144–145.

St Hill, P., Lipson, J., & Meleis, A. (2003) *Caring for women cross-culturally.* Philadelphia: F.A. Davis.

Sanchez-Bueno, F., Cuende, N., Matesanz, R. & Parrilla, P. (2005) Emergency organ transplantation in Spain: Liver emergency and outcomes. *Transplantation Proceedings* 37, 3878–3880.

Siminoff, L.A. & Sturm, C.M.S. (1998) Nursing and the procurement of organs and tissues in the acute care hospital setting. *Nurs Cl N Amer* 33(2), 239–251.

Smedley, B., Stith, A. & Nelson, A. (Eds) (2003) Unequal treatment: confronting racial and ethnic disparities in health care. Washington DC: The National Academies Press.

Solheim, K. (2005) Patterns of community relationship: nurses, non-governmental organizations and internally displaced people. *International Nursing Review* 52, 60–67.

World Health Organization (WHO) (1991) *Human organ transplantation: A report on developments under the auspices of WHO (1987–1991).* Geneva, Switzerland: WHO.

World Health Organization (WHO) (2003) *Human organ and tissue transplantation.* Geneva, Switzerland: WHO.

Yeung, I., Kong, S.H. & Lee, J. (2000) Attitudes towards organ donation in Hong Kong. *Soc Sci & Med* 50, 1643–1654.

Chapter 9
Alleviating suffering

Suffering has been defined as a state of severe distress that people experience when some crucial aspect of themselves, their being, or their existence is threatened (Cassell 1991; Kahn & Steeves 1986). It is important to understand that while there has been a tendency in the health professional literature to treat pain and suffering as being the same thing, they are not. Kahn & Steeves (1986), suggest, for example, that although suffering may be *associated* with pain – the perception of which, they argue, is usually grounded in some physical cause – suffering derives more from 'the individual's evaluation of the significance or meaning of the pain experienced', not the physical pain state itself (Kahn & Steeves 1986, p. 625). Cassell (1991) likewise suggests that while pain is a major cause of suffering, suffering *itself* is 'not confined to physical symptoms' (e.g. people can be in pain, yet not be 'suffering'). Suffering, he goes on to show, may derive from other aspects of 'personhood' – including the cognitive, emotional, spiritual, social and cultural aspects of a person's identity – not just their physical aspect. Moreover, when any one or a combination of these aspects is threatened, a person may simultaneously give a cognitive, emotional, spiritual, social, and other (cultural) meanings to that threat and respond accordingly.

Cassell explains that people frequently associated pain with suffering when:

'. . . they feel it is out of control, when the pain is overwhelming, when the source of the pain is unknown, when the meaning of the pain is dire, or when the pain is apparently without end' (Cassell 1991, p. 36).

In light of these views it can be seen why pain may or may not invoke suffering, and why threats that do not derive from a physical cause (e.g. threats to the integrity of one's personal identity) may nonetheless invoke suffering (Cassell 1991; Kahn & Steeves 1986).

Nurses deal with human suffering on a daily basis in the course of their work and have an important and fundamental role to play in alleviating the suffering encountered (Johnstone 2004; Kahn & Steeves 1986). Moreover, the relief of suffering is pivotal to protecting the human dignity of the patient and promoting the patient's good. This perhaps explains why the role of the nurse in alleviating suffering is reflected in all professional codes of nursing ethics, including the International Council of Nurses (ICN) Code (2006a). As indicated in Chapter 3, moral reasons for caring nurse behaviours include concern for how the patient is experiencing his or her world and concern for human need. Supported by the ethical principle of beneficence, nonmaleficence and justice, and the obligation to remain faithful to one's commitments, alleviating suffering is another aspect of the fundamental responsibility of the nurse.

An ethical question that often arises with this responsibility is the sometimes difficult differentiation between alleviating suffering and assisting death in seriously ill patients who are at the end stage of life. Easing the suffering of a chronically ill patient who is not at the end stage of an illness or near death may not pose ethical questions for the nurse. However, when faced with the suffering of a seriously ill patient who is at the end stage of life, nurses may experience ethical conflict between their responsibility to alleviate patient suffering and the moral obligation not to take human life. The following case example explores this conflict in the care of a seriously ill patient whose suffering is increasing as she nears death.

Case example 15: How far should the nurse go in alleviating suffering?[1]

What is the story behind the value conflicts?

Mary P was a 38-year-old woman who had recently been diagnosed with acute myelomonocytic leukaemia. Mrs Sapountzi, the nursing supervisor of the oncology unit, was present when Mary's physician, Dr T, informed Mary of her condition. Dr T presumed that Mary would want to begin chemotherapy treatment immediately. However, after learning that this form of leukaemia was successfully cured in only 25% of cases, even after extensive treatment, Mary asked to go home to discuss the entire matter with her family, her mother and an older sister.

Mrs Sapountzi called Mary the next day and learned that she did not seem to want chemotherapy for her condition. The manager of a small clothing store owned by her family, Mary had been seriously ill with cervical cancer ten years ago, had suffered from several bouts of depression and had recently had a total hysterectomy. Now 38 years old, she valued her close-knit family, their lifestyle and family-owned business. Weary of daily battles with physical and emotional ailments, she felt this new illness was quite unfair. She agreed to meet with Mrs Sapountzi and Dr T in two days' time to discuss her options.

During the meeting, Mary was adamant about not wanting chemotherapy, preferring to live whatever time she had left outside the hospital as much as possible. She was convinced that she would probably suffer terrible pain and anguish during the treatment, would be hospitalised most of the time, and would probably lose control over her body. Mary asked whether the oncology staff would help a suffering patient to die when the end was near. Dr T told Mary that physician-assisted suicide was not legal in their country although he personally did not object to helping a patient die. Mrs Sapountzi sympathised with Mary and her concerns, explaining again and again how the nurses cared for patients undergoing chemotherapy for this condition and the kind of supportive care she could expect if treatment were not successful. In the end, however, the nurse supported Mary's ultimate decision to forgo treatment because there was no way that she could assure Mary that all the things she feared would not occur. In fact, Mrs Sapountzi clearly remembered that of the three patients with acute leukaemia most recently cared for on their unit, all had experienced painful and protracted deaths (she did not tell Mary this).

Over the next few months, Mrs Sapountzi saw Mary several times when she visited the hospital for tests and minor procedures. She developed a close relationship with Mary, calling her once or twice a week to check on her mental outlook and condition. One day Mary confided to Mrs Sapountzi that when the time came that she could no longer maintain control over her life or the pain of her disease had become unbearable, she wanted to be able to take her life in the least painful way possible. She had discussed this with her mother and sister and, although they respected her decision, they thought they could not actively assist her to die. Mary asked the nurse for information about organisations that supported euthanasia so she could learn how to take her own life. Mrs Sapountzi asked Mary to make an appointment with Dr T to talk things over with him and to visit with her as well. She informed Dr T about the questions that Mary was asking.

Two weeks later, Mary had an appointment with Dr T and obtained from him the names of three organisations that supported euthanasia. Talking with Mrs Sapountzi after the appointment, she asked the nurse many questions about barbiturates, other pain medications and their effects on the body. She told the nurse that Dr T had given her a prescription for barbiturates as she was having trouble falling asleep at night and another prescription for a potent pain medication. Mrs Sapountzi made sure Mary knew how to use the medications for pain and sleep. However, she suspected that Mary was beginning to save up medications for ending her life when the time came. When she discussed the matter with Dr T, he agreed with her suspicions.

Over the next few months, Mary remained in fair condition though several serious infections and their treatments left her weak and very thin. Mrs Sapountzi arranged home nursing visits to Mary as fever, bone pain and chronic fatigue began to dominate her life. Dr T and Mrs Sapountzi suspected that the end was approaching. On Mary's last visit to the clinic, the young woman had clung to Mrs Sapountzi's hand, thanked her for being so good to her during her illness, and said 'goodbye' several times.

Two days later, Mary's sister called to say that Mary had died. She had said final goodbyes to her family and then asked her mother and sister to leave her alone for a while. After several hours, they returned to the apartment to find her dead on the living room couch; she was wearing her favourite dress and seemed at peace. They had no doubts about the course of action she had chosen. They called the family physician rather than an ambulance and he pronounced her dead from her leukaemic condition. No autopsy was performed.

Since Mary's death, Mrs Sapountzi often wonders whether nurses or physicians should help patients to end their lives in the face of severe suffering. She also wonders why a sensitive patient like Mary had to spend her final hours alone and take her own life. She knows that she and the nursing staff could have lessened Mary's suffering toward the end and provided love, comfort and care during her final moments. But they could not have completely eliminated Mary's suffering and the pain that she would have endured. Although neither Mrs Sapountzi nor Dr T directly assisted Mary in her suicide, they each helped indirectly to make it possible and as relatively painless as possible. How far should a nurse really go in alleviating patient suffering?

What is the significance of the values involved?

Attitudes toward euthanasia and physician-assisted suicide have changed dramatically over the past decade, although acceptance of these related practices varies significantly across and even within different countries (Cohen et al. 2006; De Beer et al. 2004; Dupuis 2003; Johnstone 2004; Magnusson 2002; Oehmichen & Meissner 2000; Teisseyre et al. 2005). Although public opinion in several nations is broadly supportive of euthanasia (defined as the intentional termination of a patient's life by a physician, upon the request of that patient), it has been legalised in only two countries (The Netherlands in 2001 and Belgium in 2002) (Daverschot & van der Wal 2001; De Beer et al. 2004; Dupuis 2003; Johnstone 2004). Although euthanasia was legalised in the Northern Territory of Australia in 1995, the euthanasia law (which came into force 1 July 1996) was overturned by the Australian Federal Government in March 1997, just eight months after it had come into effect (De Beer et al. 2004; Johnstone 2004). Physician-assisted suicide, in turn, has been legalised in only one jurisdiction, notably in the US state of Oregon (Sullivan, Hedberg & Fleming 2000); the Oregon legislation, however, continues to face staunch resistance and 'attack' by political conservatives in that country (Magnusson 2002, p. 64).

In most western countries, withholding and/or withdrawing life-sustaining measures at the end stage of life in order to allow a patient to die (deemed by some to be a form of 'passive' euthanasia) is both widely accepted and practised. Nonetheless there are those both within and outside the healthcare professions who advocate the public acceptance and legalisation of euthanasia (Johnstone 2004). There are at least two reasons for this support. First, it is believed that acceptance would bring an existing practice 'out of hiding'. Claiming that euthanasia is already being practised by many physicians and nurses in some countries, they believe that public acceptance would encourage discussion about the practice and would help to establish formal criteria upon which decisions to perform euthanasia should be based (Crock 1998; Kevorkian 1991; Magnusson 2002; Quill 1993).

Second, public acceptance of euthanasia would help establish acceptable procedures for euthanasia, make it available for all citizens, and take the decision out of the hands of private individuals who otherwise have no standards of accountability to the public or in the public arena (Lach 1990). This would prevent potential abuses of euthanasia and ensure that the decision for euthanasia was based on sound reasoning rather than rhetoric (Lanham 1993).

Others, however, adamantly oppose the role of any health professional – especially nurses – in the euthanasia or assisted suicide of patients (Berghs et al. 2005; Daverschot & van der Wal 2001; De Beer et al. 2004; Keown 1995). They claim that such involvement is incompatible with the fundamental role of the health provider, including nurses (Kopala & Kennedy 1998; Zimbelman 1994; Zimbelman & White 1999). Critics particularly worry that, if the practice became widespread and the role of nurses in participating in euthanasia practices was given legal recognition, patients might lose trust in nurses (Johnstone 1996). Others further claim that acceptance of active euthanasia could weaken society's commitment to provide care for the terminally ill and dying (Johnstone 2004; Uhlmann 1998).

What is the significance of the conflicts to the parties involved?

Assisted suicide occurs when a patient requests assistance in dying from someone else, often a healthcare worker, but performs the lethal act themselves (Johnstone 1996, 2004). Although assisted suicide was once viewed as inconsistent with the professional role, the news media report that increasing numbers of health providers provide assistance to individuals faced with a debilitating (but not necessarily end stage) illness who want to end their lives. Healthcare workers' participation in acts of euthanasia and requests for assistance to suicide are usually related to mercy and the relief of patient suffering (Crock 1998; Fry & Veatch 2006; Teisseyre et al. 2005). However, should any healthcare worker assist in putting a suffering patient out of his or her misery by hastening their death, with or without their consent? This is the moral question that Mrs Sapountzi faced in caring for her patient, Mary P.

What should be done?

Historically, codes of nursing ethics have been ambiguous about what actions nurses should or should not take when confronted with the possibility of euthanasia or assisting a patient with his or her suicide, especially a patient who is suffering from an end stage illness and is in intractable pain (Johnstone 1996, 2004; Berghs et al. 2005; Seymour et al. 2007). Nurses have a responsibility to alleviate suffering, to relieve pain and to make any patient as comfortable as possible. But does nursing responsibility extend to assisting a patient to die? If the patient is no longer physically able to carry out his or her wishes to die, should the nurse, perhaps, even kill the patient, in other words, commit an act of euthanasia?

Unless the role of the nurse is clarified in legislation, the answer to both of these questions is 'No'. The nurse's responsibility to alleviate suffering does not mean to eliminate suffering by ending the patient's life. Nurses have a responsibility to take all reasonable means to protect and preserve human life when there is hope of recovery or reasonable hope of benefit from life-prolonging treatment. During the dying process, and in keeping with the codified ethical standards of the profession, nursing care should always be directed toward the compassionate prevention and relief of suffering (ICN 2006a, 2006b). However, some nursing measures used to relieve symptoms in the dying patient may entail substantial risk of hastening death. These measures are designed to relieve suffering and pain, not to bring about the death of the patient. If the patient does die while these measures are being used in his or her care, the nurse is not necessarily morally responsible for the patient's death or for using the measures. If in doubt about the moral dimensions of any nursing actions with a patient suffering from an end stage illness or a patient who is requesting assistance with suicide, the nurse should always be familiar with the guidelines of the nursing association of his or her country, institutional or agency policies and the moral guidelines for the practice of nursing worldwide.

Case example 16: Alleviating the dehumanisation and suffering of elderly patients

What is the story behind the value conflicts?

T Skoldjck is a new graduate nurse providing nursing care to elderly patients in a hospital ward. Few relatives visit the patients so she has little knowledge of the lives these patients enjoyed prior to becoming dependent on others for their care. Some of the patients are semi-comatose but many seem to be aware of their surroundings and can respond to verbal commands. They wander the halls, calling out for former friends or loved ones, wring their hands while walking, cry and look miserable. Those confined to their beds moan whenever anyone comes near and clutch at the person in a desperate manner. Some cry out in a pleading voice, 'Please, I want to die.'

Because there is limited staff to care for these patients, all of them are treated in a similar manner. A team of three nurses enters the ward every two hours either to feed, bathe or turn the bedridden patients in an assembly-line fashion. The patients are kept clean and dry. Their medications and a liquid supplement are often supplied by nasogastric tubes, despite the fact that a few of the patients are capable of taking nourishment by mouth. Patients who can get out of bed are tied in chairs and given a glass of juice. When finished with the juice, they are ushered back into bed for a rest period.

Miss Skoldjck is troubled by the way nursing care is being provided to these patients but does not know what to do. She is reluctant to criticise the care plans that have been designed by other, more experienced nurses, particularly when patients receive regular physical care. She wonders, however, why the chronically ill and bedridden patients do not seem to have the same basic human rights to privacy, protection of human dignity and alleviation of suffering that younger and less debilitated patients seem to have. How should a nurse alleviate the suffering of these elderly patients?

What is the significance of the values involved?

According to the UNFPA (2005), over the next 45 years, the number of persons in the world aged 60 years or older is expected to almost triple, increasing from 672 million people in 2005 to nearly 1.9 billion by 2050. Of these people, it is anticipated that 80 per cent will be living in developing countries, and 20 per cent in developed countries. Currently, in developed countries, just one-fifth of the population is 60 years or older; by 2050, however, this proportion is expected to rise to almost a third (UNFPA 2005). Meanwhile, those who are 80 years old or over (the 'oldest old'), are expected to increase from 86 million in 2005 to 394 million in 2050. By 2050, most oldest-old people (the majority of whom will be female) will be living in the developing world (UNFPA 2005).

Over the past two decades, elderly patients in many countries have become the most vulnerable, disadvantaged individuals in the healthcare system (Binstock & Post 1991; Moody 1992). Improved nutrition and better healthcare have greatly extended the average lifespan of older people (Chiva & Stears 2001). Yet the joys of living well and living longer are not always experienced by many elderly people today. Some of the elderly are simply not in good health and must depend on others for support and care. If they have poor health, they require a larger proportion of healthcare resources and social services during their final years than ever before (Daniels 2006).

Some elderly individuals have no immediate family or relatives to provide housing, care or financial and emotional support (Nay & Garratt 2004). Many live alone or in institutions that seem designed to meet the needs of the caregivers rather than the needs of the elderly themselves (Edwards et al. 2003). In some countries, a large portion of the elderly live in poverty or near-poverty conditions. Many (especially those with debilitating ailments) give up on life as evidenced by international data indicating that older people, worldwide, are at a higher risk than any other age group of completed suicide (Lester & Tallmer 1994; O'Connell et al. 2004).

What is the significance of the conflicts to the parties involved?

The questions that Miss Skoldjck has about the care of elderly patients on her ward are not uncommon. Nurses have long experienced many ethical conflicts in the care of institutionalised and often demented elderly patients (Norberg, Asplund & Waxman 1987). Nurses are responding to these questions and the situation of the elderly by demanding that the specific needs of the elderly be recognised (ICN 2006b). At the very least, healthcare systems and related resource allocations need to adapt to the growing numbers of elderly who require nursing care support (Daniels 2006; Nay & Garratt 2004). They need to propose and initiate new models of care for the healthy elderly in residential communities (WHO 2004). Such models would foster the self-determination of elder citizens and provide protection of their dignity and privacy during their remaining years. With assistance, many elderly can live long and meaningful lives. With appropriate living arrangements, many can manage activities of daily living as they age.

What should be done?

Where the needs of Miss Skoldjck's patients are concerned, care must be taken to ensure that they are treated respectfully. Their human needs for companionship, touch, comfort and relief of pain and suffering can be satisfied by appropriate nursing measures. Many elderly patients confined to bed do not experience enough attention and human contact to keep them oriented to the present time and place. Left alone for long periods of time without communication and positive human interaction, their minds wander to past events and past relationships, often making them appear senile. Nursing attention to elderly patients' particular needs for human contact can do much to alleviate their loneliness and loss of orientation. Offering human touch and conversation to elderly patients often helps them to consume food and take in fluids. Merely placing a glass of juice in front of an elderly patient does not convey much beyond recognition that he or she is a biological entity that requires calories in order to continue living. Surely our elderly citizens deserve more recognition and attention than this?

The International Council of Nurses supports the role of nurses in the planning of care for the elderly in its Position Statement *Nursing Care of the Older Person* (2006c). This statement indicates that the aim of nursing care with the elderly is to help them to achieve optimal health, well-being and quality of life. Nurses are encouraged to participate in their nursing associations' efforts to influence health policy in their countries so that care that enhances the dignity of the elderly is available to all who need it. The elderly should not be singled out in any country to receive the lowest cost or standard of care simply because they are old.

Everyone has the right to seek asylum and to find refuge in another country, with the option to return voluntarily to their country of origin when conditions permit or to resettle in another land (UNHCR 2002). Over the past five decades, an estimated 50 million people across more than 116 countries have been assisted to 'restart their lives' either as refugees or internally displaced people (UNHCR 2002). It has been conservatively estimated that, currently, there are approximately 25 million internally displaced and refugee peoples in the world (ICN 2006d). The health status of these people is often poor, rendering them particularly vulnerable and in need of help to find and adjust to a new way of life (ICN 2006d).

* * * *

The responsibility to alleviate suffering extends to nurses caring for those who are escaping armed conflict and torture in their home countries, who have become displaced persons, and/or who have become political refugees (Glittenberg 2003; ICN 2006d; Welch & Welch 2000). These persons often represent a challenge to nursing care because much of their suffering is emotional and psychological, as well as physical. They have often witnessed the destruction of their homes, their communities and their family members, and may have been tortured themselves. Their suffering may follow cultural patterns unfamiliar to nurses working with relief services and to those from other cultures. However, nurses have an important role in addressing the health needs of refugees and civilian populations (ICN 2006d). The following case example explores how one nurse struggled with her responsibility to alleviate suffering while serving as a nurse volunteer with a church-supported relief service in a distant country.

Exercise:

Case example 17: The silent refugee

S Duffy is a white European nurse who is working in a refugee camp in Asia. For months, the camp has taken in 10–50 refugees each day since bitter fighting broke out among religious fundamentalists in a neighbouring state. Rumours of torture have recently drifted in with the refugees but no actual torture victims have been identified. Miss Duffy, however, suspects that Puli, a young girl of about 16 years of age who was carried in by a refugee family several weeks ago, has suffered mistreatment of some kind. The girl keeps herself wrapped in a shawl and refuses a physical examination when Miss Duffy asks her about some strange marks on her thighs and upper back. She never talks, and she walks with a shuffling gait as if her feet hurt. When Miss Duffy tries to talk to Puli, the girl becomes very alarmed and moves away from her. She absolutely refuses to allow the male physician to touch her body. Should Miss Duffy force a physical examination on the refugee's body? How can she relieve her physical suffering if Puli won't allow her to assess its extent and nature?

Discussion questions

What is the story behind the value conflicts?

(1) What is the ethical problem confronting Miss Duffy where her nursing practice is concerned?

(2) What are the values involved from Miss Duffy's perspective? From Puli's perspective?

What is the significance of the values involved?

(3) Postulate the meanings of Miss Duffy's values to her. Of Puli's values to Puli.

(4) Are there any professional value questions posed by this situation involving questions of nursing care to Puli?

What is the significance of the conflicts to the parties involved?

(5) Which values held by Puli and Miss Duffy seem to be in conflict?

(6) How do Puli's values affect Miss Duffy's nursing practice?

(7) How do Miss Duffy's values affect Puli's sense of well-being?

(8) If Miss Duffy forces her nursing attention on Puli, what might be the probable outcomes of such action?

(9) If Miss Duffy leaves Puli alone in her suffering, what might be some of the probable outcomes of this action?

What should be done?

(10) What is Miss Duffy's ethical responsibility to Puli in this situation?

(11) What ethical actions should Miss Duffy take in caring for Puli? Why?

(12) Is it possible for Miss Duffy to honour her professional values and respect Puli's values at the same time as providing care for Puli? Why or why not?

(13) What guidelines would you offer for nurses caring for refugees that would help them to know what is ethical nursing practice under these conditions? Why?

Summary

The realities of everyday nursing practice often force the nurse to seriously reconsider his or her ethical responsibilities. While the professionally mandated ethical responsibility to alleviate suffering is clear, acting on this responsibility may not be easy when the patient is at the end stage of life, elderly or recovering from an unusual and tragic human event. People experience human suffering in different ways and with different abilities to deal with their suffering. The nurse's responsibility to alleviate suffering means that the nurse must carefully assess the suffering of any patient and carefully gauge the patient's internal resources for coping with suffering. Nursing care to alleviate the patient's suffering will then be specific to the individual and the type of suffering experienced.

Note

1 Adapted from Quill, T.E. (1991) Sounding board: Death and dignity. *NEJM*, 324(10), 691–694.

References

Berghs, M., Dierckx de Casterlé, B. & Gastmans, C. (2005) The complexity of nurses' attitudes toward euthanasia: a review of the literature. *Journal of Medical Ethics* 31(8), 441–446.

Binstock, R. & Post, S. (Eds) (1991) *Too old for health care? Controversies in medicine, law, economics, and ethics*. Baltimore: Johns Hopkins University Press.

Cassell, E. (1991) *The nature of suffering and the goals of medicine*. New York: Oxford University Press.

Chiva, A. & Stears, D. (Ed) (2001) *Promoting the health of older people*. Buckingham: Open University Press.

Cohen, J., Marcoux, I., Bilsen, J., Deboosere, P., van der Wal, G. & Deliens, L. (2006) European public acceptance of euthanasia: socio-demographic and cultural factors associated with the acceptance of euthanasia in 33 European countries. *Social Science & Medicine* 63(3), 743–756.

Crock, E.A. (1998) Breaking (through) the law – coming out of the silence: nursing, HIV/AIDS and euthanasia. *AIDS Care* 10(2), S137–145.

Daniels, N. (2006) Equity and population health. *Hastings Center Report* 36(4), 22–35.

Daverschot, M. & van der Wal, H. (2001) The position of nurses in the new Dutch Euthanasia Bill: a report of legal and political developments. *Ethics & Medicine* 17(2), 85–91.

De Beer, T., Gastmans, C. & Dierckx de Casterlé, B. (2004) Involvement of nurses in euthanasia: a review of the literature. *Journal of Medical Ethics* 30(5), 494–498.

Dupuis, H. (2003) Euthanasia in the Netherlands: 25 years of experience. *Legal Medicine* 5(Suppl. 1), S60–S64.

Edwards, H., Courtney, M. & O'Reilly, M. (2003) Involving older people in research to examine quality of life in residential aged care. *Quality in Aging* 4(4), 38–43.

Fry, S.T. & Veatch, R.N. (2006) *Case studies in nursing ethics*, 3rd ed. Boston: Jones & Bartlett Publishers.

Glittenberg, J. (2003) The tragedy of torture: a global concern for mental health nursing. *Issues in Mental Health Nursing* 24, 627–638.

International Council of Nurses (ICN) (2006a) *Code of ethics for nurses*. Geneva, Switzerland: ICN.

International Council of Nurses (ICN) (2006b) *Position statement: Nurses' role in providing care to dying patients and their families*. Geneva, Switzerland: ICN.

International Council of Nurses (ICN) (2006c) *Position statement: Nursing care of the older person*. Geneva, Switzerland: ICN.

International Council of Nurses (ICN) (2006d) *Position statement: Health services for migrants, refugees and displaced persons*. Geneva, Switzerland: ICN.

Johnstone, M.-J. (Ed) (1996) *The politics of euthanasia: A nursing response*. Deakin, ACT: Royal College of Nursing, Australia.

Johnstone, M.-J. (2004) *Bioethics: a nursing perspective*, 4th ed. Sydney: Harcourt Saunder.

Kahn, D. & Steeves, R. (1986) The experience of suffering: conceptual clarification and theoretical definition. *Journal of Advanced Nursing* 11(6), 623–631.

Keown, J. (Ed) (1995) *Euthanasia examined: Ethical, clinical and legal perspectives.* Cambridge, UK: Cambridge University Press.

Kevorkian, J. (1991) *Prescription: Medicide: The goodness of planned death.* Buffalo, NY: Prometheus Books.

Kopala, B. & Kennedy, S.L. (1998) Requests for assisted suicide: A nursing issue. *Nurs Ethics* 5, 16–26.

Lach, J. (1990) Active euthanasia. *J Clin Ethics* 1(2), 113–115.

Lanham, D. (1993) *Taming death by law.* Melbourne: Longman Professional.

Lester, D. & Tallmer, M. (1994) *Now I lay me down: Suicide in the elderly.* Philadelphia: Charles Press.

Magnusson, R. (2002) *Angels of death: Exploring the euthanasia underground.* Melbourne: Melbourne University Press.

May, W.F. (1982) Who cares for the elderly? *Hast Ctr Rep* 12(6), 31–37.

Moody, H. (1992) *Ethics in an aging society.* Baltimore: Johns Hopkins University Press.

Moody, H.R. (Ed) (1994) *Aging: Concepts and controversies.* Thousand Oaks, CA: Pine Forge Press.

Nay, R. & Garratt, S. (Eds) (2004) *Nursing older people: Issues and innovations*, 2nd ed. Sydney: Elsevier/Churchill Livingstone.

Norberg, A., Asplund, K. & Waxman, H. (1987) Withdrawing feeding and withholding artificial nutrition from severely demented patients: Interviews with care givers. *WJ Nurs Res* 9(3), 348–356.

O'Connell, H., Chin, A., Cunningham, C. & Lawlor, B. (2004) Recent developments: suicide in older people. *British Medical Journal* 329, 895–899.

Oehmichen, M. & Meissner, C. (2000) Life shortening and physician assistance in dying: Euthanasia from the viewpoint of German legal medicine. *Gerontology* 46, 212–218.

Quill, T.E. (1993) *Death and dignity.* New York: W.W. Norton and Co.

Seymour, J., Janssens, R. & Broeckaert, B. (2007) Relieving suffering at the end of life: Practitioners' perspectives on palliative sedation from three European countries. *Social Science & Medicine* 64(8), 1679–1691.

Sullivan, A.D., Hedberg, L. & Fleming, D.W. (2000) Legalized physician-assisted suicide in Oregon: The second year. *NEJM* 342, 598–604.

Teisseyre, N., Mullet, E. & Sorum, P. (2005) Under what conditions is euthanasia acceptable to lay people and health professionals? *Social Science & Medicine* 60(2), 357–368.

Uhlmann, M.M. (Ed) (1998) *Last rights: Assisted suicide and euthanasia debated.* Grand Rapids, MI: Eerdmans.

UNFPA (2005) *Fast facts: Population issues.* New York: United Nations Population Fund.

United Nations High Commission for Refugees (UNHCR) (2002) *Refugee resettlement: An international handbook to guide reception and integration.* Geneva, Switzerland: UNHCR.

Welch, T. & Welch, M. (2000) Listening for the sounds of silence: A nursing consideration of caring for the politically tortured. *Nursing Inquiry* 7, 136–141.

World Health Organization (WHO) (2004) *A glossary of terms for community health care and services for older persons.* Geneva, Switzerland: WHO.

Zimbelman, J. (1994) Good life, good death, and the right to die: Ethical considerations for decisions at the end of life. *J Prof Nurs* 10(1), 22–37.

Zimbelman, J. & White, B.C. (1999) The moral appeal of assisted suicide in end-of-life decisions. *J Prof Nurs* 15(3), 142–145.

Part 3
Applying ethics to nursing practice

Applying ethics to nursing practice can be influenced by various personal, professional, social, cultural and political factors. Codes of nursing ethics help define ethical nursing practice by providing broad guidelines for nursing actions under ideal conditions. Codes of nursing ethics, however, are not designed to provide easy answers to complex ethical questions that might be raised in different healthcare situations. These codes do not tell the nurse what she or he should do in caring for a specific patient. To decide what action one ought to take in caring for a specific patient, the nurse must apply knowledge of ethics within the context of the situation at hand.

The International Council of Nurses (ICN) *Code of Ethics for Nurses* (2006) indicates that the nurse's fundamental responsibilities – to promote health, prevent illness, restore health and alleviate suffering – extend to all health services offered to the individual, the family groups and the community. In addition to these fundamental responsibilities, nurses also have specific responsibilities. First, nurses have a primary responsibility to respect the values and to protect the privacy of the people who require nursing care. Second, by working cooperatively with other health professionals, the nurse takes responsibility to protect the patient's health from unsafe practices. Third, by working cooperatively with other citizens, nurses take responsibility to initiate and support actions designed to meet the health needs of the public.

Finally, nurses have personal and professional responsibility to maintain their competence in practice and to uphold high standards of nursing care. By maintaining standards of professional conduct in practice situations, the nurse reflects credit upon the profession.

Part 3 explores the nature of nursing responsibility as outlined in the ICN *Code of Ethics for Nurses* (2006) in relation to people, nursing practice, the profession and co-workers in healthcare. Ethical principles (Chapter 2), ethical concepts (Chapter 3), and the Model for Ethical Analysis and Decision Making in Nursing Practice (Chapter 5) are applied to case examples in each chapter. The scope of nursing responsibility in relation to the people served by nursing care is explored in Chapter 10. Subsequent chapters apply ethics to the nature of nursing practice (Chapter 11), to the profession of nursing (Chapter 12) and to the nurse's co-workers (Chapter 13). Actual patient care examples demonstrate the ethical responsibility of the nurse in a variety of situations involving complex bioethical issues.

Chapter 10
Nurses and people

The International Council of Nurses (ICN) *Code of Ethics for Nurses* states that the nurse's primary responsibility is to 'people requiring nursing care' (2006a, p. 2). In providing care, the nurse 'promotes an environment in which the human rights, values, customs and spiritual beliefs of the individual, family and community are respected'. The nurse then 'holds in confidence personal information and uses judgment in sharing this information' with others. These statements define the ethical dimensions of nursing responsibilities to the people that nurses serve.

Who are the people who require nursing care? Do we assume that ALL citizens and non-citizens (e.g. residents, refugees, asylum seekers, and internally displaced persons) require nursing care at some time or another? Or does nursing only serve those people who seek out nursing care? Do nurses have a responsibility to those who could benefit from nursing care but are currently outside the healthcare system? Answering these questions will help us understand to whom nurses have a primary responsibility and how the nurse provides needed care in a just manner.

Serving people who need nursing care

Nurses generally care for more than one patient at a time. In some cases, patient needs will be equal in their importance or severity and the nurse will have to choose which needs should be met first. In other cases, the recognition of patient needs will be influenced by external factors (such as access to healthcare or ability to pay) and may result in some patients' needs not being met. The following patient care situation demonstrates one kind of ethical conflict nurses experience in providing nursing care.

Case example 18: Are some patients more important than others?

What is the story behind the value conflicts?

Fawzi K was a nurse in a small city that was attacked by hostile military forces from a neighbouring country. Her small hospital received many wounded soldiers from her country's military forces during the first 24 hours of battle. As the city was overtaken, soldiers from the invading forces were also brought to the hospital for emergency treatment. Ms K and the other nurses did not really want to take care of the invaders and wondered if they were obliged to do so. The wounds of the enemy soldiers were severe and in some cases life-threatening. Yet Ms K found it difficult to provide care to them, especially when soldiers of her country also needed medical attention. Since the small hospital had only limited medical supplies, the physicians in charge quietly told each nurse to allocate primary attention and supplies to the national troops and provide only comfort measures, including pain relief, to the foreign soldiers. They were also to care for all soldiers before giving attention to wounded civilians. Ms K agreed that their own soldiers should receive the best treatment possible but she wondered if it were ethical, all things considered, to distribute medical supplies in this manner. Under conditions of armed conflict, should physicians and nurses decide who is more needy of services than others? Are soldiers more worthy of treatment than civilians?

What is the significance of the values involved?

The duties of medical and nursing personnel are explained in the Geneva Conventions of 1949 and their Additional Protocols (Astrada 1982) (Figure 10.1). All persons, prisoners of war and civilians exposed to the consequences of an armed conflict are protected by the provisions of international humanitarian law (ICN 1999). This means that they must be treated humanely under all circumstances. In addition, medical and nursing personnel have certain 'special obligations' that derive from their professional standards of ethical conduct and which must be fulfilled. They should not be punished for having discharged their medical/nursing functions in keeping with medical/nursing ethics nor should they be compelled to act contrary to their professional ethics.

However, all citizens value their freedom, their way of life, their country and its customs. Whether one is a nurse or a physician, these values are important to them as citizens. Any citizen would want to help the armed forces of their own

---

1.1   Medical personnel who provide their services in armed conflicts must respect the principles of medical ethics in the same manner as in peacetime.

1.2   Persons who do not take a direct part in hostilities and those placed 'hors de combat' shall be treated humanely.

1.3   Care must be given without any distinction based on other than medical criteria.

1.4   It is prohibited to subject protected persons to any medical procedure which is not indicated by their state of health and to carry out on them any medical, biological, or other scientific experiments.

1.5   The will of the wounded and sick must be respected.

1.6   Reprisals against protected persons and objects are prohibited.

Figure 10.1   Duties of medical personnel during armed conflict: The provision of medical care (Adapted from Astrada 1982, pp. 36–43).

Position statement – The nurse's role in the care of detainees and prisoners

Nurses' primary responsibility is to those people who require nursing care. In caring for detainees and prisoners nurses are expected to adhere to ethical principles and the following:

- Nurses who have knowledge of abuse and maltreatment of detainees and prisoners take appropriate action to safeguard their rights.
- Nurses employed in prison health services do not assume functions of prison security personnel, such as body searches for the purpose of prison security.
- Nurses participate in clinical research on prisoners and detainees only with the prisoner or detainee's informed consent.
- Nurses collaborate with other health professionals and prison authorities to reduce the impact of crowded and unhealthy prison environments on transmission of infectious diseases such HIV/AIDS and tuberculosis.
- Nurses abstain from using their nursing knowledge and skills in any manner which violates the rights of detainees and prisoners.
- Nurses advocate for safe humane treatment of detainees and prisoners including clean water, adequate food and other basic necessities of life.

Figure 10.2 Excerpts from the ICN Position Statement (ICN 2006c).

country. While they might not want to harm the invaders, it is understandable that caregivers would want to give every possible advantage to their fellow citizens. This sentiment can cause a troubling conflict between professional and personal values when the health professional must care for soldiers of both sides of an armed conflict at the same time.

What is the significance of the conflicts to the parties involved?

The International Council of Nurses' Position Statement: *The Nurse's Role in the Care of Detainees and Prisoners* (2006c) states its support of the Geneva Conventions and specifically states that 'prisoners and detainees have the right to health care and humane treatment; also a right to clear and sufficient information to refuse treatment or diagnostic procedures; and to die with dignity and in a peaceful manner' (p. 1) (Figure 10.2). Nurses are expected to provide nursing care to anyone injured in an armed conflict, friend or foe, by giving unbiased attention to their injuries and by making sure that no one is subjected to cruel, inhumane or degrading treatment. To fail in this responsibility is unethical behaviour.

Now, it might seem that the ethical principles of beneficence and non-maleficence – the obligations to do good and to avoid harm – should primarily guide the nurse in making an ethical decision under conditions of armed conflict. However, the simple balancing of good versus harm is not an acceptable moral standard for this type of situation. Deciding what is good or harmful may vary among nurses and some might even consider it good (or, at least, not harmful) to allow the enemy soldiers to die. Surely it might be considered good to attend to one's own soldiers before enemy soldiers. While balancing good versus harm may be important in deciding how one cares for soldiers of both sides during an armed conflict, the principles of beneficence and nonmaleficence alone do not provide adequate moral direction for why the nurse should provide care in a just and equitable manner to all injured soldiers and citizens.

The requirements of the Geneva Convention and the ICN's Position Statements *Armed Conflict: Nursing's Perspective* (1999) and *The Nurse's Role in the*

Care of Detainees and Prisoners (2006c) are supported by the ethical principle of justice and the ethic of care. As we learned in Chapter 2, the principle of justice means that nurses must decide how their nursing resources ought to be distributed among patient populations. The nurse must ask: What is a fair allocation of my nursing care resources among all the patients under my care? As discussed in Chapter 3, following an ethic of care means that one considers the duties of the relationship (injured soldier and nurse) and strives to avoid hurting others (nonmaleficence) as well as oneself. Self-interested motives are avoided while care toward others is promoted.

In times of armed conflict, any soldier should expect that justice and care principles, not personal values or preferences, will guide attention to the injuries suffered on the battlefield. This is a minimal expectation for the health needs of all soldiers in time of war and is supported by the mandates of organisations such as the International Committee of the Red Cross (ICRC). As part of their professional role, nurses are also expected to be compassionate in providing care to all injured parties during an armed conflict.

What should be done?

While it might seem easy to provide needed nursing care as directed by the physicians, each nurse must decide what he or she ought to do according to his or her own assessments of moral and professional obligations in the situation. Each nurse should be familiar with the requirements of the Geneva Conventions of 1949 and their Additional Protocols. These documents serve to protect soldiers and citizens during the special situation of armed conflict. The nurse should also be familiar with the standards of the nursing profession and with the expectations of professional nurses as outlined by the International Council of Nurses and other organisations. During times of doubt and uncertainty, these standards serve as guides for the nurse's actions.

Even with these considerations about armed conflict, the nurse must finally decide which patient has the greatest need and focus the majority of his or her time on that patient. If the nurse decides to provide care in a just and equitable manner to all armed personnel, he or she will still need to decide where professional skills can have the most benefit. Obviously, the amount of good that is done will vary depending on the intensity of the need. Some nurses will consider physical needs of greater importance than psychological needs. If that is the case, then determining the amount of benefit received by the patient might prove difficult. Psychological needs are harder to quantify than physical needs. How much consideration should Fawzi K give to patient needs in deciding who her patients are?

Considering that the needs of the injured soldiers may be different from the needs of the citizens, Ms K will need to determine which injuries are more life threatening and proceed from there. If the nurse decides to give his or her attention according to need and uses supplies according to need, he or she will be providing care in an ethical manner congruent with the moral and legal requirements of international humanitarian law. All injured soldiers and citizens will be treated humanely and nurses, in turn, will not be punished later for carrying out their professional ethics during time of war. As the ICN (1999, p. 1) points out, 'nurses have an important role to play in addressing the impact of emergency and long term health needs of refugees, other civilian populations and wounded armed forces personnel and demands protection for all health professionals providing care and relief personnel in conflict zones'.

Individual versus collective good

A fundamental tension often exists between the nurse's obligation to benefit the individual patient and the obligation to benefit society. Sometimes the individual nurse must decide whether her primary obligation is to promote individual good or to promote collective good. The following patient care situation demonstrates how one nurse experienced this tension between the two kinds of good.

Case example 19: Promoting individual good at high financial cost[1]

What is the story behind the conflict?

Felicitas M is a 6-year-old child with acute leukaemia. She has had several relapses while on chemotherapy. The specialist suggests that a bone marrow transplant is the only treatment that offers Felicitas a reasonable hope of survival. This procedure is very costly and Felicitas receives only public assistance for her healthcare. She would need to go to a larger city 160 miles away and stay there for many months while being treated. The treatment does not offer a total cure for the leukaemia, either. The estimated cost of the treatment will use more than two-thirds of the budget usually allotted to children with debilitating diseases in this whole health district.

Felicitas' mother and father ask the nurse in charge of the clinic services to help them process their request for the treatment. They ask her how to move their child's name higher on the waiting list for the procedure. What should she say to them? Should the nurse make a judgment on how much 'doing good' for this patient costs or the possible expense to other children?

What is the significance of the values involved?

Nursing supports both the value of individual good and the value of collective good. The ICN *Code of Ethics for Nurses* indicates that the nurse 'promotes an environment in which the human rights, values, customs and spiritual beliefs of the individual, family and community are respected' (2006a, p. 2). Service to the individual, however, is emphasised by statements such as, 'The nurse ensures that the individual receives sufficient information on which to base consent for care and related treatment' (p. 2). The value of collective good, or the good of society, is supported by statements such as, 'The nurse also shares with society the responsibility for initiating and supporting action to meet the health and social needs of the public, in particular those of vulnerable populations' (p. 2). It is clear that the nurse is expected to promote both the individual good and the collective good.

Felicitas M's nurse will want to promote the individual good of her young patient. This is an important moral value. However, she will probably consider the individual good of other children who might have substantial healthcare needs as this is also her professional responsibility. The nurse values providing the best possible care for Felicitas but may consider the benefits to Felicitas against as yet unknown but potential benefits of healthcare services to other children over time. The nurse also values the authoritative role of parents in making decisions for their child.

The parents of Felicitas surely value the health of their child and cannot be expected to consider the healthcare needs of any other child. They have an obligation to their child and it is not reasonable to expect them to want anything except what is best for Felicitas.

Society, however, does not look at individual needs and whether individual patients could benefit from specific treatments. Society only values serving the greatest number of citizens with whatever healthcare resources are available. This means that individual needs and benefits may be overlooked in distributing resources to the greatest number. Which of these values should receive first priority?

What is the significance of the conflicts to the parties involved?

Ethical nursing practice means providing services for the benefit of the individual patient, the patient already in a relationship with the nurse. In the case of Felicitas, if more good can be done by spending funds allotted to child health on her personal care than on any other person's care, then supporting this choice would amount to a convergence of the nurse's clinical commitment to advocate for this patient and the promotion of overall good using society's resources. Even so, there still would be a conflict over whether it is fair for one person (Felicitas), even though she is very ill, to have such a disproportionate share of the available monies spent on her needs.

If the money is to be spent for those who have the greatest need, Felicitas must surely be considered because her need is great. But if there is to be some balance between individual need and collective need, then it would seem that Felicitas is receiving more than her share. Some adjustment between these values will have to be made.

It might be argued that more overall good could be achieved for more people if the money needed for Felicitas' care was divided among several people. But should the nurse make this kind of decision if Felicitas is her patient? There seems to be a fundamental problem of professional ethics when nurses begin to consider whether they should benefit the patient before them with the resources at hand or consider how much good they could do for other unknown people if they distribute their resources differently. This is not the type of decision that healthcare workers really want to make and, quite possibly, not the kind that they ought to make. If the nurse were removed from giving direct care to Felicitas and her parents, perhaps it would be possible for her to decide more objectively whether to promote individual good at the expense of the collective good. But that is not the case with Felicitas' nurse. She has a relationship with an individual patient that seems to preclude making decisions for the collective good when doing so will compromise the individual good of this patient.

What should be done?

The nurse in this situation can help Felicitas' parents weigh the benefits of treatment against the potential harms of having no treatment as they wait for their request for treatment to be processed. There is no guarantee that Felicitas will receive the bone marrow transplant. Even if the health district authorises the cost of the treatment, the family must wait for a suitable donor. The likelihood of finding a donor is slight and Felicitas and her parents must be prepared for this outcome. The nurse does not have the option of making a decision for or against the treatment as this decision will occur outside her realm of influence. Discussing this type of issue in professional and public meetings, however, offers nurses an opportunity to help formulate policies and guidelines for these types of decisions. The nurse will always consider the needs and rights of the patient already under her care as having first priority. But there may be instances when some needs are so great that they take priority over all other needs, even those of patients already under the care of the nurse. Collaboration and cooperation in making this type of decision may be necessary for the nurse to consider adequately how to balance the collective good with an individual good.

Respecting values, customs and spiritual beliefs

Nurses often care for individuals who have value orientations very different from their own. This may create values conflicts for the nurse trying to do good for the patient, especially when the patient's cultural definition of good differs from the nurse's definition of what is good for the patient's health. The customs that individuals follow in speaking about illness and their spiritual beliefs may also influence the kind of nursing measures that are designed and implemented in patient care. Yet nurses are expected to create a caring environment in which patients' values, customs and spiritual beliefs are respected. Is the nurse held responsible for everything that may occur within the healthcare environment that can potentially affect the patient? Certainly not. Nurses, as the most constant healthcare contact with patients and families, have a responsibility to select healthcare resources that will be conducive to a therapeutic environment for the patient, but they are not necessarily responsible for developing these resources. Nevertheless, nurses are responsible for the decisions they make within this environment.

In the following patient care situation, the nurse experiences ethical conflict while trying to create an environment where the patient's values, customs and spiritual beliefs are respected.

> **Case example 20: Is it ethical to override religious beliefs to preserve life?**[2]
>
> ### *What is the story behind the value conflicts?*
>
> C Adade, a nurse midwife, practises in a 280 bed district hospital in a central African country. One day a 24-year-old woman, pregnant with twins, is admitted in premature labour to the birthing unit. She has received her prenatal care in another district and is unknown to the hospital staff. The patient's haemoglobin is found to be very low (4.7 mg) so preparation for blood transfusion is made. At this point the patient states that she is a Jehovah's Witness and will not consent to any blood transfusion. Mrs Adade talks to the patient's husband, hoping that he will encourage his wife to consent to the transfusions. However, he agrees with his wife in refusing blood products. Mrs Adade respects the choices of the couple but calls a physician to assist in what she thinks might become a difficult delivery situation.
>
> Within the hour the first twin is born and appears to be in good condition. The patient, however, begins to show signs of cardiac failure and becomes unresponsive. Mrs Adade feels that she ought to do whatever she can to save the life of the unborn twin so she starts the transfusion shortly before the physician arrives. The second child is born and requires resuscitation which eventually proves successful. The mother, however, goes into complete cardiac failure even though she has

received three units of blood. Attempts to resuscitate her are unsuccessful and she dies in the birthing unit. Following the birth, the physician tells Mrs Adade that starting the blood transfusion was the appropriate thing for her to do. He does not think it necessary to tell the husband that his wife received blood transfusions during the delivery but he leaves this decision to her. Did Mrs Adade do the right thing? Should she tell the husband that the wife received blood transfusions before she died?

What is the significance of the values involved?

Mrs Adade is a nurse midwife who respects the choices and values of her patient. When her patient said that she could not consent to a blood transfusion because of her religious beliefs Mrs Adade respected this choice and called a physician for what she suspected would be a difficult birth. She wanted to protect her patient and the unborn children from harm insofar as possible. However, when faced with the failing condition of the young woman and the resulting decreased supply of oxygen to the unborn twin, Mrs Adade's moral values (to preserve life) and professional values (to prevent harm) conflicted with her respect for the beliefs and values of the patient.

As a member of Jehovah's Witnesses, the young mother espouses a set of religious beliefs forbidding the blood transfusion. Jehovah's Witnesses are known for refusing this type of treatment based on their interpretation of Scriptural prohibitions against the 'eating of blood' (Watch Tower Bible and Tract Society of Pennsylvania 1977; see also Johnstone 2004; McInroy 2005; Stroup 1987). Although the young mother undoubtedly did not want to die and did not want to harm her unborn children as a result of refusing treatment, she could not conscientiously consent to the blood transfusion due to the strength of her religious beliefs.

What is the significance of the conflicts to the parties involved?

The ICN *Code of Ethics for Nurses* clearly claims that the nurse has a moral responsibility to promote 'an environment in which the human rights, values, customs and spiritual beliefs of the individual, family and community are respected' (2006a, p. 2). Mrs Adade provided this environment when she accepted the patient's refusal of the blood transfusion. However, consideration for the unborn twin and his right to life conflicted with the mother's right to refuse this treatment. In western legal cases involving the right of a Jehovah's Witness patient to refuse blood transfusions, the courts usually respect the choice of the adult Jehovah's Witness patient (McInroy 2005). However, when the interests of children are involved, the courts usually override the parents' refusals and order that medical treatment, including blood transfusions, be given to the children. This is because the courts consider the life of a child to be of greater value than the parents' right of refusal based on religious belief.

Jehovah's Witnesses themselves recognise that when children are involved, the issue of refusing a life-saving blood transfusion is one that is 'most highly charged with emotion' (Watch Tower Bible and Tract Society of Pennsylvania 1977, p. 33). A foundational and long-standing position of the Jehovah's Witnesses is stated:

> 'All of us realize that children need care and protection. God-fearing parents particularly appreciate this. They deeply love their children and keenly feel their God-given responsibility to care for them and make decisions for their lasting welfare' (Watch Tower Bible and Tract Society of Pennsylvania 1977, p. 33).

In regard to doctors administering blood to a child against the expressed wishes of the parents, they state:

'Frankly, in view of the well-recognized right of parental responsibility, the moral, principled and consistent position for a doctor is to recognize the responsibility of loving, concerned parents to make decisions for their minor children' (Watch Tower Bible and Tract Society of Pennsylvania 1977, p. 35).

To do otherwise, they argue, is to perpetuate a position that 'lacks fundamental consistency and harmony' and that violates the religious rights of children that are otherwise accorded to the adults of the Jehovah's Witness faith (Watch Tower Bible and Tract Society of Pennsylvania 1977, p. 35). They further assert that doctors and the courts recognise the rights of adult Jehovah's Witnesses to refuse blood transfusions.

Contrary to popular belief, if a life-saving blood transfusion is given to a child against the wishes of parents (say, for example, by court order), the child will not be ostracised by fellow Jehovah's Witnesses. While Jehovah's Witnesses do sanction members who wilfully and deliberately disobey established religious doctrine (sanctioning can take the form of religious counselling and/or, in serious cases of deviant conduct, formal ostracisation or 'disfellowship' of the offending member for periods of time that can range from months to years), this only applies to those who have been baptised into the faith (Botting & Botting 1984; Penton 1985). Baptism, in accordance with Jehovah's Witnesses doctrine, is a ritual that is not performed on children. Only those who have attained the age of 'maturity' and who can make a reasoned choice to commit themselves to the faith are encouraged to be baptised (Botting & Botting 1984; Penton 1985). Thus, children who receive blood transfusions without parental consent will not be ostracised. To the contrary, such children are likely to be seen as the 'victims of medical assault', will receive extraordinary support from their brethren, be viewed as having been maligned by the 'old order' or 'evil world', and may even be treated as martyrs and praised and supported accordingly. Likewise with adults who have been given blood transfusions against their will – for example, being given a life-saving blood transfusion while unconscious (Johnstone 2004).

Acting to promote the mother's choices could be supported by the ethical principle of autonomy. However, since the life of the child is in question, the prevention of harm (nonmaleficence) to the child and the preservation of the mother's life to prevent harm to the child could be seen to outweigh the requirement to respect patient autonomy in this case – although this calculation is by no means without controversy. Thus, Mrs Adade's actions to initiate the blood transfusion would be supported by the ethical principles of nonmaleficence and fidelity. Following the delivery of the twins and the death of the mother, however, Mrs Adade finds that she must now make another ethical decision – whether to tell the husband about the blood transfusion. The physician tells Mrs Adade that telling the husband is not necessary, probably because he does not want the husband to find fault with the birthing and the procedures employed. He leaves the decision of whether to tell the husband up to Mrs Adade.

Not to tell the husband is an act of deception. Both he and his wife refused the blood transfusion and he believes that this wish was respected by Mrs Adade. One might argue that the most caring thing to do for the grieving husband would be not to add to his grief and worries. Any adult Jehovah's Witness patient might be troubled by the fact that a blood transfusion was used in treatment. Such patients often believe that receiving a blood transfusion violates God's commands and thus places on them an enormous burden of suffering (Botting & Botting 1984; Penton 1985; Watch Tower Bible and Tract Society of Pennsylvania 1977), even though responsibility for giving the transfusion belongs to the healthcare team. Would it not be more caring to simply not tell about the transfusions to avoid troublesome outcomes for the husband and the children?

What should be done?

It can be argued that Mrs Adade should not deceive the husband or withhold information from him about the blood transfusion. She respected the couple's choices until the life of the child was endangered. She is obliged to respect the values, customs and spiritual beliefs of all individuals who receive nursing care. However, she is also responsible for her practice and must use her judgment in providing care. In this situation, her judgment was to save the life of the child if at all possible without risking the life of the patient. Based on this reasoning, her actions of starting the transfusion when she did could be seen to be justified by appealing to the moral principle of nonmaleficence – although just how this principle ought best to be interpreted remains an open question. The principle of veracity (the obligation to tell the truth and not to lie or deceive) would support that she must inform the husband about the blood transfusion. The father has a right to know that blood products were used during the birth of his children. Respect for his spiritual beliefs and values would lead to telling him about treatment that conflicts with these beliefs and values, with the nurse and the physician taking responsibility for the treatment decision. This knowledge would also enable him to seek appropriate support from his brethren within the Jehovah's Witness faith.

Protecting human rights and dignity

The need to safeguard human rights is universal. Protecting basic human rights, especially human dignity, creates special responsibilities for the nurse (McHale & Gallagher 2003). When these responsibilities conflict with other values and rights believed to be important, ethical questions arise.

The threat to human rights knows no geographic boundaries. Armed conflicts occur in many countries, creating political upheaval, anarchy, starvation and mistreatment of many human beings. People are detained for political or criminal reasons, resulting in potential threat to their basic human rights. Wherever nurses practise, they have a responsibility to safeguard the rights of people who are being physically or mentally abused, tortured or who have life-sustaining healthcare withheld from them. They must also be aware of more subtle ways in which people may be degraded, abused or otherwise deprived of basic human rights. The ICN Position Statement *Nurses and Human Rights* (2006b) (Figure 10.3) makes it clear that nurses are accountable for their own professional actions and must be alert to the possibility of being pressured to use their knowledge and skill as a nurse in a manner that is not truly beneficial to patients or others (Johnstone 1988).

Position statement – Nurses and human rights

The International Council of Nurses (ICN) views health care as a right of all individuals, regardless of financial, political, geographic, racial or religious considerations. This right includes the right to choose or decline care, including the right to accept or refuse treatment or nourishment, informed consent; confidentiality, and dignity, including the right to die with dignity. It involves both the rights of those seeking care and the providers.

Nurses have an obligation to safeguard and actively promote people's health rights at all times and in all places. This includes assuring that adequate care is provided within the resources available and in accordance with nursing ethics. As well, the nurse is obliged to ensure that patients receive appropriate information in understandable language prior to consenting to treatment or procedures, including participation in research.

Nurses are accountable for their own actions and inactions in safeguarding human rights, while National Nurses Associations (NNAs) have a responsibility to participate in the development of health and social legislation related to patient rights.

Where nurses face a 'dual loyalty' involving conflict between their professional duties and their obligations to their employer or other authority, the nurse's primary responsibility is to those who require care.

Figure 10.3   Excerpts from the ICN Position Statement (ICN 2006b).

Violations of basic human rights often occur during times of political upheaval. Degradation of prisoners, starvation, torture and mass killings of ethnic minorities are not uncommon. Torture is defined as 'the systematic and deliberate infliction of acute pain in any form by one person on another or on a third person, in order to accomplish the purpose of the former against the will of the latter' (Tornbjerg & Jacobsen 1986). Should nurses avoid any contact with prisoners whom they suspect have been tortured? Certainly not. The nurse's primary responsibility is to those who require nursing care (see Figure 10.4). If the nurse sees a prisoner who has been victimised or tortured and who requires nursing care, then the nurse is obliged to give such care to the best of his or her nursing ability. The nurse should also know how to report torture to appropriate national and/or international bodies without fear of personal retribution (Rueda-Castanon 1998; Tornbjerg & Jacobsen 1985).

Torture occurs in many situations, not all of them political. Torture of patients can occur whenever healthcare workers act violently toward a patient for other than therapeutic reasons. The mental sequelae of being tortured, in any form, are great (Dind 1989).

Survivors of torture sometimes fear healthcare workers because such workers were present when they were tortured or advised how the torture should be carried out for the greatest physical effect. These survivors often experience depression, extreme fatigue, loss of sexual functioning, headaches and recurring nightmares about their imprisonment or torture sessions. Many bear excessive guilt feelings from being forced to watch the torture of friends and loved ones (Glittenberg 2003; Jacobsen & Vesti 1989; Racine-Welch & Welch 2000; Rasmussen 1990; Solheim 2005).

Position statement – Torture, death penalty and participation by nurses in executions
The International Council of Nurses strongly affirms that nurses should play no voluntary role in any deliberate infliction of physical or mental suffering and should not participate, either directly or indirectly, in the preparation for and the implementation of executions. To do otherwise is a clear violation of nursing's ethical code of practice.

The nurse's primary responsibility is to those people who require nursing care.

Nurses have a duty to provide the highest possible level of care to victims of cruel, degrading and inhumane treatment, and should speak up against and oppose any deliberate infliction of pain and suffering.

While ICN considers the death penalty to be unacceptable, clearly the nurse's responsibility to a prisoner sentenced to death continues until execution.

ICN believes that all levels of nursing education curricula should include recognition of human rights issues and rights to refuse to participate in executions; violations, such as torture and death penalty; awareness of the use of medical technology including lethal injections for executions; and recognition of the nurse.

Figure 10.4   Excerpts from the ICN Position Statement (ICN 2006d).

The following case example demonstrates the ethical conflict experienced by one nurse in caring for a political detainee whom she suspected was being tortured.

Exercise:

Case example 21: Caring for a political prisoner

What is the story behind the conflict?

B Ortiz, a health clinic nurse, and the clinic physician have been brought to a camp where political detainees are confined. The nurse and physician have been here before to treat minor ailments among the prisoners. Last month they advised hospitalisation of two prisoners with symptoms of kidney injuries whom they believed had been tortured. This month, they are being asked to do physical assessments and histories on several new prisoners. The first prisoner is taken away as soon as his examination is complete. An hour later, he is returned to the examining room unconscious. He has multiple contusions on his face, missing teeth, a dislocated jaw and a noticeably swelling elbow. Several of his fingers have been broken or the joints dislocated. The physician and nurse treat his wounds after determining that he does not have any life-threatening injuries. Several days later, on another visit to the compound, the physician/nurse team notices the man lying in an adjoining shed. He appears to be very seriously injured and is having trouble breathing. The guards tell them to forget about this prisoner and simply treat the other ones. Ms Ortiz is concerned that if the man does not receive immediate attention, he may stop breathing and die. What should she do? Should she provide care to the prisoner even though it will make the guards angry? Should she refuse to do health assessments on the new prisoners for fear that they might be treated likewise? Will she suffer harm if she does not cooperate with the guards?

Discussion questions

What is the significance of the value conflicts involved?

  (1) What are the values being expressed by Ms Ortiz?

  (2) What are the values being expressed by the guards of the camp?

  (3) What do you presume to be the values and human rights of the unconscious prisoner?

  (4) Are there any professional or legal standards that might guide nursing responsibility in this case? What are they?

  (5) Which values seem to be in conflict?

What is the significance of the conflicts to the parties involved?

  (6) What makes the value conflicts significant to the parties involved?

  (7) What are the policy guidelines that might need to be changed or created as a result of this situation?

  (8) What is the likelihood that the nurse or her family (if she has one) will suffer harm if she does not cooperate with the camp director? And what bearing could and should this have on her decision making?

  (9) How might her actions affect the particular prisoner's health? The health of the other prisoners?

What should be done?

 (10) What potential actions might Ms Ortiz take in the situation?

 (11) Should she provide care to the prisoner even though this will probably make the guards angry and may also place her own life and well-being at risk? Should she refuse to do further health assessments on the other prisoners? Should she refuse to come to the camp in the future?

 (12) Which of the available options open to the nurse are morally permissible? Which options are not morally permissible?

 (13) If you were Ms Ortiz, what would you do?

Ms Ortiz has a legitimate concern that prisoners are being tortured in the camp she is visiting. Although she and the clinic physician are not directly participating in any acts of torture themselves, they are assisting in the physical examinations of prisoners prior to their being subjected to torture. They are also being asked to assist in treating the effects of torture, making it possible for further interrogations involving torture to take place. While it is clear that nurses should not participate in, or be present during, torture of human beings under any circumstances, it is not clear whether providing first aid treatment may create the opportunity for further acts of torture when the prisoner's condition improves (Johnstone 1988; Nightingale & Chill 1995).

    Many refugees of political upheaval find their way to other countries, bringing with them major healthcare needs that present challenges to healthcare workers in the adopted country (Kemp 1993). Nursing care for victims of torture always requires respectful treatment, understanding and sensitivity. If possible, nursing care should be delivered in quiet places with privacy. When the environment, such as a prison camp, does not allow these resources, the nurse must exercise care and prudence in treating the injured person. Learning about the provision of nursing care under such conditions is seldom part of basic nursing education but opportunities for this kind of preparation should be available to any nurse who may confront the effects of torture. When persons have been abused or tortured, nursing care should focus on physiological and psychological support of the patient and the family, emphasising physical and emotional security as well as nutritional intake (Randall & Lutz 1991; UNHCR 2002). Such an approach is supported by the ethical principles of beneficence, nonmaleficence, justice and fidelity and by the ethic of care discussed in Chapters 2 and 3.

Summary

Nursing responsibilities to the people whom nursing serves can often conflict with other values and professional expectations. Protecting human rights and patient dignity can be difficult when others decide that some patients are more worthy of nursing time and attention than others. Honouring the spiritual beliefs, customs and values of patients can also create ethical tension when these values conflict with professional duties. Providing nursing care for the survivor of torture will be especially difficult in a country experiencing political reform or upheaval. Each situation requires the nurse to examine the nature of the nurse's primary responsibility to the people needing care in the context of the ethical requirements of professional practice.

Notes

1　Adapted from Fry, S.T. & Veatch, R.M. (2006) *Case studies in nursing ethics*, 3rd ed. Boston: Jones & Bartlett, Publishers (p. 81). Used with permission.
2　Adapted from Tate, B.L. (1977) *The nurse's dilemma: Ethical considerations in nursing practice*. Geneva: ICN (p. 15). Used with permission.

References

Astrada, A.B. (1982) *Manual on the rights and duties of medical personnel in armed conflicts*. Geneva, Switzerland: International Committee of the Red Cross.
Botting, H. & Botting, G. (1984) *The Orwellian world of Jehovah's Witnesses*. Toronto: University of Toronto Press.
Dind, C. (1989) Teaching nurses about torture. *Intl Nurs Rev* 36(3), 81–82.
Glittenberg, J. (2003) The tragedy of torture: A global concern for mental health nursing. *Issues in Mental Health Nursing* 24, 627–638.
International Council of Nurses (ICN) (1999) *Position statement: Armed conflict: Nursing's Perspective*. Geneva: ICN.

International Council of Nurses (ICN) (2006a) *Code of ethics for nurses.* Geneva, Switzerland: ICN.

International Council of Nurses (ICN) (2006b) *Position statement: Nurses and human rights.* Geneva: ICN.

International Council of Nurses (ICN) (2006c) *Position statement: The nurse's role in the care of detainees and prisoners.* Geneva: ICN.

International Council of Nurses (ICN) (2006d) *Position statement: Torture, death penalty and participation by nurses in executions.* Geneva: ICN.

International Council of Nurses (ICN) (2006e) The nurse, the Geneva Conventions, and human rights. *Intl Nurs Rev* 39(2), 61–63.

Jacobsen, L. & Vesti, P. (1989) Treatment of torture survivors and their families: The nurse's function. *Intl Nurs Rev* 36(3), 75–80.

Johnstone, M.-J. (1988) Support for Amnesty International: A nursing perspective. *Australian Nurses Journal* 18(3), 10–11.

Johnstone, M.-J. (2004) *Bioethics: A nursing perspective*, 4th ed. Sydney: Harcourt/ Saunders.

Kemp, C. (1993) Health services for refugees in countries of second asylum. *Intl Nurs Rev* 40(1), 21–24.

McHale, J. & Gallagher, A. (2003) *Nursing and human rights*. London, UK: Butterworth/Heinemann.

McInroy, A. (2005) Blood transfusion and Jehovah's Witnesses: The legal and ethical issues. *Br J Nurs* 14(5), 270–274.

Nightingale, E.O. & Chill, J.C. (1995) Torture. In W.T. Reich (Ed) *Encyclopedia of bioethics*, 2nd ed. (pp. 26515–26569). New York: Macmillan.

Penton, M. James (1985) *Apocalypse delayed: The story of Jehovah's Witnesses*. Toronto: University of Toronto Press.

Racine-Welch, T. & Welch, M. (2000) Listening for the sounds of silence: A nursing consideration of caring for the politically tortured. *Nursing Inquiry* 7, 136–141.

Randall, G. & Lutz, E.L. (1991) *Serving survivors of torture: A practical manual for health professionals and other service providers.* Washington, DC: American Association for the Advancement of Science.

Rasmussen, O.V. (1990) Medical aspects of torture. *Danish Med Bull* 37(1), 1–88.

Rueda-Castanon, C. (1998) The special rapporteur on torture: Some issues relating to coordination with human rights mechanisms. *Human Rights* 3, 14–17.

Solheim, K. (2005) Patterns of community relationship: Nurses, non-governmental organizations and internally displaced persons. *International Nursing Review* 52, pp. 60–67.

Stroup, H. (1987) Jehovah's Witnesses. In M. Eliade (Ed) *Encyclopedia of Religion*, vol. 7 (pp. 564–566). New York: Macmillan.

Tornbjerg, A. & Jacobsen, L. (1985) Violation of human rights and the nursing profession. *Intl Nurs Rev* 32(6), 178–180.

Tornbjerg, A. & Jacobsen, L. (1986) Violation of human rights and the nursing profession. *Intl Nurs Rev* 33(1), 6–8.

United Nations High Commission for Refugees (UNHCR) (2002) *Refugee resettlement: An international handbook to guide reception and integration.* Geneva: UNHCR.

Watch Tower Bible and Tract Society of Pennsylvania (1977) *Jehovah's Witnesses and the question of blood.* New York: Watchtower Bible and Tract Society of New York/International Bible Students Association Brooklyn.

What health care workers should know about torture. (1990) *Intl Nurs Rev* 37(5), 326.

Chapter 11
Nurses and practice

The practice of nursing entails many ethical responsibilities. As indicated in Chapter 3, ethical concepts such as advocacy, accountability/responsibility, cooperation and caring provide a moral foundation for nursing practice. These concepts shape the ethical dimensions of the nurse's work with individuals, family groups and communities and are the basis of formal standards for nursing practice throughout the world.

The International Council of Nurses (ICN) *Code of Ethics for Nurses* (2006) contains ethical standards for nursing practice which state that the nurse 'carries personal responsibility and accountability for nursing practice and for maintaining competence by continual learning' (p. 2). When acting in a professional capacity, the nurse 'at all times maintains standards of personal conduct which reflect well on the profession and enhance public confidence' (p. 3). Whether involved in patient care or any other area of nursing practice, the nurse 'maintains a standard of personal health such that the ability to provide care is not compromised' (p. 3).

The nursing profession has a fundamental responsibility to 'contribute to health planning and policy, and to the coordination and management of health services' (ICN 2000a). When accepting and delegating responsibilities, the nurse is to use 'judgment regarding individual competence' (ICN 2006, p. 3). National nurses associations, meanwhile, have a responsibility 'to promote professional practice models that support the appropriate delegation of nursing care to assistive personnel' (ICN 2000b). This includes ensuring that the 'role, preparation, standards, and practice of assistive nursing personnel [are] defined, monitored, and directed by Registered Nurses' (ICN 2000b).

In this chapter, these ethical standards for nursing practice are explored in relation to allocating nursing care to individuals, family groups and communities, in delegating nursing authority to others and in accepting responsibility for nursing care. Nursing practice examples demonstrate the types of ethical conflicts that nurses experience in practice, and the process by which they can resolve these conflicts.

Allocating nursing care

Nurses allocate (or distribute) nursing care services in response to human need in a manner that is respectful of and does not disadvantage or discriminate against people on the grounds of a person's cultural, social or economic status or other personal attributes. The following case example demonstrates some of the ethical questions that arise in allocating nursing care resources to individuals.

Case example 22: Serving the patient whose care costs the least amount of money[1]

What is the story behind the value conflicts?

Sheila C practises nursing in a country that has recently begun to ration health-care services based primarily on costs. As the nurse practitioner in a rural clinic, she can no longer refer all patients for diagnostic testing and medical attention as she had in the past. Even though she knows that certain neurological tests, for example, may help her to provide the most appropriate care for a particular group of patients and may prevent complications, she can no longer send these patients for this service because of the costs. Other less expensive services are readily available; however, they are not as accurate and are not 'state of the art' technology. Miss C is particularly troubled that rehabilitative services for elderly patients and for those with long-term chronic diseases have virtually disappeared from medical insurance coverage. Yet these services often offer the greatest benefit to patients and prevent further deterioration of their health. She finds that she is beginning to view patients not as individuals who can benefit from her care but as 'allowable services'. The result is that some patients are getting more of her attention than others, based on factors that have nothing to do with their health-care needs. She does not believe that she is providing ethical nursing care.

What is the significance of the values involved?

Considering the basic responsibilities of the nurse (to promote health, prevent illness, restore health and alleviate suffering) does not really help Miss C to decide how much time, nursing attention and healthcare resources to allocate to her patients. She knows that she has an ethical responsibility to do good for her patients and to prevent them from being harmed. However, she also has a responsibility to use resources wisely and not increase the financial burden of the healthcare system. She wants to practise nursing in a way that reflects favourable credit upon the nursing profession without lowering the standards of nursing practice, especially during times of healthcare rationing. She must balance her obligation to uphold public welfare with her obligation to uphold the patient's welfare.

Patients, on the other hand, expect that the nurse and other health professionals will give them the best care possible. Any patient, given a choice between a highly accurate test that is costly and a less accurate test that is not as expensive, would probably choose the more accurate test regardless of cost. If the test can lead to a more accurate diagnosis, they would rather have it performed if possible. In times of healthcare rationing, however, not all tests will be available for all patients. Some patients, because of their age, will not be offered treatments using costly technologies. Other patients may not be offered costly rehabilitative services if there is little hope that they can return to a productive life. If the goal is to provide healthcare where it will benefit the most people at the least cost to the public, some services will simply not be available to all citizens in the society.

What is the significance of the conflicts to the parties involved?

If the nurse decides that doing the most good is her primary responsibility, then she might choose to care for patients who can most benefit from her own set of unique nursing skills. This approach to patient care will lead to very subjective judgments which may not be fair. In fact, the criteria that one nurse uses to determine good may well differ from that of another nurse. One nurse might think preserving life is the highest good. Another might think that the ability to return to a productive life is the highest good. A third nurse might think that freedom from pain is the highest good, and so on. This is the type of decision that Miss C might make if she decides to consider patient good as the most important factor in providing nursing care to her patients.

If serving patient good is not the goal, then the nurse might decide to give patients equal amounts of available resources because that is the most equitable thing to do. Since the needs of patients are different, however, the amount of good that would occur would vary among patients. Does the amount of good done to patients really matter if all are served equally? Some nurses would argue that treating patients equally is ethically preferable to deciding which patient can benefit the most from nursing care. But again, equal treatment does not seem to be the ethical question that concerns Miss C.

Miss C is concerned about the cost of healthcare since cost eventually affects everybody served by the healthcare system. Certainly, there is room for concern about healthcare costs – by governments, legislators, policy makers and the like. Professional nursing organisations also should play a strong role in determining cost-effective and quality nursing care. In addition, there needs to be greater recognition by all concerned of the positive impact that quality nursing care can have on patient outcomes and indeed on the cost-effectiveness of healthcare generally, and how these outcomes might best be measured (Aiken et al. 2003; Christensen et al. 2000; Kurtzman & Kizer 2005; Needleman et al. 2002; Page 2004). Determining the quality of patient care on the basis of cost, however, is not an easy task. Here the important question arises: should nurses consider the cost of care in deciding how to allocate nursing care among individual patients? This is the ethical question faced by Sheila C as she practises nursing within a healthcare system that rations services based on costs.

What should be done?

The first decision in considering whether to refer patients for costly diagnostic services is establishing the priorities for the distribution of available healthcare services at the macro or policy/healthcare system level (Kilner 1995a). This is accomplished by policy makers, legislators and government officials on behalf of and with the community they serve. Health promotion, prevention of illness or health maintenance are often some of the priorities involved (Daniels 2006; Powers & Faden 2006).

A second decision concerns the most effective and efficient method to allocate available resources. Should the emphasis be placed on direct healthcare services (clinics and programmes) or should indirect services (health education and clinic transportation services) receive a higher (or equal) emphasis?

A third decision involves establishing the appropriate relationship between rescue services and preventive services within the healthcare delivery system. Should the majority of resources be concentrated on critical care services? Or should the major focus of nursing effort and resources be prevention of disease and disability through, for example, childhood immunisation and well baby visits.

Fourth, a decision is made as to which diseases or categories of illness take precedence over others in the attention they are given by health workers. For example, should the prevention and treatment of HIV infection take precedence over the prevention and treatment of breast cancer? Decisions made on precedence can result in allocating significant financial and nursing resources to certain socioeconomic or racial groups and must be carefully considered in their full context to avoid ethical conflicts.

Finally, in establishing certain priorities, it is important to consider whether or not these priorities compromise important values and principles held by the community or even by the professional group. For example, preventive strategies aimed at discouraging alcohol consumption or smoking may emphasise behavioural or lifestyle changes by members of the community. Priority setting in relation to lifestyle can have a substantial impact on the autonomy of community members and may conflict with their social, cultural or religious values. Priority setting may also conflict with the nurse's professional values. Miss C suspects that her country's healthcare rationing strategies are beginning to compromise her professional values and her obligation to maintain high standards of nursing care. Once the priorities for allocating healthcare resources to all citizens are established, nurses and other healthcare professionals will need to decide who will receive their services and what criteria will be used to determine who gets what. This is making healthcare allocation decisions at the micro level or at the level of individual care (Kilner 1995b).

Criteria frequently used to allocate nursing services after determining patient need include deciding who will benefit most from the nurse's expertise and the cost of giving that care. Miss C seems to be working with this type of decision. She will need to decide how relevant these criteria are to the patients' needs, the ethical requirements of nursing practice and the continuing role that nursing might have in the care of each patient. Guided by the ethical principles of beneficence, nonmaleficence and justice, immediate ethical questions about the healthcare rationing scheme might be resolved (Beauchamp & Childress 2001). At the level of individual patient care recommendations, these principles provide direction for decision making in similar situations. The ethic of care and its focus on the nurse–patient relationship help provide direction for decision making in individual patient care situations. However, the ethic of care alone will not be an adequate guide during times of cost containment when healthcare resources must be rationed (Johnstone 2004).

Delegating nursing authority to others

Nurses need to exercise great care in how they delegate patient care to others. The nurse's ethical responsibility and accountability for the quality of care does not end simply because the patient care task or tasks are delegated. In deciding when and to whom to delegate patient care, the nurse needs to consider the education, knowledge and capabilities of the person to whom care is delegated, the severity and complexity of the patient's condition, the available supervision for the care delivered and the nature of nursing care required. The following case demonstrates ethical questions that arise when nurses are asked to delegate nursing functions to non-nurses.

Case example 23: Accountability for delegated responsibilities[2]

What is the story behind the value conflicts?

Ivan G is Director of Nursing of an 80-bed nursing home for elderly people in a small urban community. He has been involved with other nursing home administrators, district health officers and physicians in an effort to provide cost-effective but high quality healthcare services for elderly citizens in their city. He suddenly learns that legislation has been introduced in the provincial government that will allow unlicensed personnel in nursing homes to administer all medications. Ivan G is quite concerned. As an advocate of skilled nursing care in nursing homes, he knows that administering medications to elderly people is much more than merely giving ordered dosages of chemical substances. The administration of medications is an important part of nursing home care. For medications to be effective in maintaining and improving the health of the elderly, they must be administered by licensed nursing personnel who can monitor the effects of those medications on the patients.

Although the law has permitted unlicensed personnel to give medications in province-owned psychiatric hospitals for many years, the nursing association has been working to change this practice. The nursing association has argued that the administration of medicines in nursing homes and psychiatric hospitals is a nursing function which must be performed by licensed nurses. Now, it seems the policy makers in the provincial government are directly challenging the professional organisation on this position.

After a few telephone calls, Ivan G learns that the legislation was introduced by a politician who supports a group of businessmen who want to build a nursing home facility in his home district. The businessmen have argued that unlicensed personnel, if properly trained and supervised, can do the same job as licensed nurses. Their work will present no real risk to elderly people in nursing homes and will, in the long run, be more cost-effective since the salaries of licensed nurses have risen dramatically in the last few years. The proposed legislation has the support of the provincial pharmaceutical association and other politicians. What can Ivan G and his nursing colleagues do to halt the passage of this legislation?

What is the significance of the values involved?

To Ivan G and his nurse colleagues, the health of elderly people in nursing homes is an important professional value. They believe that licensed nurses are best qualified to administer medications to the nursing home residents and to monitor the effects of medication in each person. In their opinion, unlicensed personnel cannot be held accountable for their practice and cannot be expected to skilfully assess the health of elderly patients whose needs are often complex. Administration of medications is simply not a function for unlicensed personnel.

To the politician and the group of businessmen, providing custodial care at the least cost is the highest value. This will be good for the public (the least amount of taxes) and good for their own pockets (increased profits) and will not pose a significant risk to elderly people themselves. Whatever risk is involved is judged insignificant in comparison to the cost savings that will result.

To the elderly residents, having the best care possible at the least amount of cost to them is the highest value. Since they have already worked and contributed to societal good, they feel entitled to nursing home care that protects their safety and promotes their well-being and human dignity.

What is the significance of the conflicts to the parties involved?

The need for nursing participation in the political process is quite evident in this situation. Three issues seem to be creating ethical conflicts on different levels.

The first issue is the quality of patient care in nursing homes and the potential risks of adverse events to nursing home residents if medications are administered by unqualified or unlicensed personnel (Fry & Veatch 2006). For Mr G and his nurse colleagues, this is the basic value conflict. If the legislation is passed, as professional nurses they will be directly responsible for the medication admin- istration expertise in their institutions, even though they do not administer the medications themselves. They will then be in the uncomfortable position of being responsible for a practice not only that they disagree with, but over which they have no legitimate authority (Johnstone 1994).

The second issue in this situation involves the kinds of trade-offs one can be comfortable with in achieving cost-effective nursing home care. Ivan G and the nursing association take the position that high quality nursing home care requires that medications be given by licensed (or registered) nursing personnel. The politicians and businessmen are taking the position that cost-effective nursing home care means replacing, in part, the high cost of licensed nurses by allowing unlicensed or unregistered personnel to give medications. The crucial question is whether the quality of nursing home care should be sacrificed for cost-effectiveness. The ethical tension between the two choices is an example of one of the most common ethical dilemmas in healthcare: doing what is right accord- ing to accepted moral standards of contact, or doing what is right according to desired financial outcomes or consequences (Fry & Veatch 2006).

The third issue concerns the profession's mandate for collaboration among members of the nursing profession, other healthcare workers and policy makers in matters concerning the delivery of healthcare. The fact that members of the community (businessmen) and another professional group (the pharmacists' association) are in support of the legislation seems to create considerable tension between collaborative efforts of nurses and others in the community to provide high quality, cost-effective nursing home care. At what point should members of one professional group feel obligated to negotiate their differences with another group? Is compromise on these types of issues ever ethically acceptable? If so, under what conditions? If not, how can tensions between professionals and community groups be resolved in order to preserve joint effectiveness on larger political issues concerning health?

What should be done?

It is clear that the profession's mandate for nurses to be involved in political issues does not adequately assess the complexity of many issues. Professional nurses might have to take a different position from that previously taken in order to create change or to wield power in the political arena that affects healthcare (Gordon 2005). To resolve this type of conflict, Ivan G and his nurse colleagues will need to be politically informed about all aspects of this particular issue and other impending issues regarded as important by the politicians and businessmen. This will require not only political understanding on their part, but research-based evidence of the possible risks and benefits of allowing medications to be administered by unqualified or unlicensed caregivers. For example, it is suspected that medication errors increase when medications are not administered by licensed or registered nurses. Ivan G and his nurse colleagues will need to provide a convincing case that this is a possibility, as well as show that the financial costs of these errors outweigh any benefits from medication administration by less costly caregivers. They can also request that stringent processes are in place to ensure that the potential of risks to elderly people in nursing homes will be kept to a minimum if and when medication practices are changed. If Ivan G and his nurse colleagues decide that compromise is not an option, then they will need to be prepared to present nursing concerns to the appropriate people. This kind of issue requires a great deal of collaboration between individual nurses and between the professional organisation and other groups in the community (Gordon 2005).

Other ethical questions can arise when patient care is delegated to others under less than optimal conditions. The following case describes the ethical questions one nurse experienced when this happened to her.

Case example 24: When nursing responsibilities seem overwhelming

What is the story behind the value conflicts?

Taka Osako is the nurse unit manager for a 15-bed critical care unit. Every bed in the unit has been occupied during the past two weeks. The nurses are beginning to experience stress and physical exhaustion from providing complex care to very sick patients over an extended period of time. They are also discouraged by the number of patient deaths: five in the past two weeks.

Ms Osako learns that one of the regular nurses must take emergency leave to care for a family member who is having major surgery. Another nurse calls Ms Osaka to say that she is ill and will probably not be able to return to work for a week. Ms Osako asks the nursing supervisor for additional personnel. The supervisor agrees to send an experienced nursing aide and a graduate nurse with limited experience in critical care to the unit, and promises to find a more experienced nurse for the unit within 48 hours.

At this point, the admitting physician calls Ms Osako about the admission of a new patient. The 38-year-old man is on a ventilator and suffering from multiple physical injuries from a motorcycle accident. The physician thinks the patient will require dialysis within the next 12 hours. Ms Osako realises that this patient will need one-to-one nursing care for the first 24 hours and close supervision for 72 hours thereafter.

Ms Osako would prefer to refuse to admit this patient but recognises that the culture and customs of her country forbid it. To accommodate the new patient, she transfers an elderly woman, who is just beginning to show signs of improvement, to another unit. This action clearly distresses the nursing staff because they believe this patient still needs the attention of the staff of the critical care unit.

Ms Osako then assigns the nursing aide and the graduate nurse to two other patients who require frequent endotracheal suctioning and careful monitoring of IV fluids so that a regular nurse can take care of the incoming patient. No one is happy with Ms Osako, least of all the graduate nurse who is terrified by the monitors and other equipment surrounding the patients assigned to her. What factors should Ms Osako consider in assigning the aide and the inexperienced nurse to these patients? How far can the nurse unit manager extend her regular nursing staff without jeopardising the quality of care provided?

What is the significance of the values involved?

Ms Osako obviously values competent nursing care for the patients under her management. She considers the needs of all patients in the unit and makes patient care assignments in order to minimise any risks of harm to them from the sudden shortage of qualified nurses. While she might sympathise with her nursing staff and realise that they are experiencing stress from the previous two weeks, she must consider the needs of the patients of greater value than the needs of any of the nurses. She is a nurse manager and is expected to make decisions for the management of the unit, some of which may not necessarily favour the needs of a particular patient or nurse. But she is not expected to object to the physician's plans to place a critically ill patient in the unit. Because she values her culture (and probably her employment), Ms Osako accommodates the physician's request rather than refusing it.

The nursing staff, on the other hand, are not happy with her patient care assignments. They value their confidence in being able to provide quality care without making mistakes due to stress and overwork. They value the recent judgments they have made in providing care to the elderly woman and they value what continued nursing attention can do to improve her condition. The graduate nurse also values being licensed, and worries that she might make a mistake that could result in her being disciplined by a nurses board and possibly even losing her licence. She is right to expect that she will be relieved from providing care that she is not adequately prepared for or experienced in giving. She does not want to harm patients nor does she want to make any mistakes that will put a patient at risk of preventable harm.

The admitting physician values competent nursing care and the availability of a critical care bed for a patient when she deems it necessary. She complies with the subservient role that nurses in her country are expected to have in relation to physicians. Such a role makes it easier for the physician to obtain the care that she believes necessary for her patients. She may also value the success of her medical treatment with this critically ill younger man more than the continued medical care of the elderly woman who is transferred to another unit.

The patients also value competent nursing care. The elderly woman who is transferred values her life and her continued improvement. However, like other women of her age in the sociocultural context in which she lives, she does not object to being transferred and simply accepts the judgment of the physician. The fact that she is a female and elderly, and gives up her bed for a young male patient is not considered as being possibly discriminatory, but as the 'right', and even altruistic, thing to do – i.e. for the good of the younger generation.

What is the significance of the conflicts to the parties involved?

Nursing practice standards provide little direction in this case situation. The ICN *Code of Ethics for Nurses* (2006) requires the nurse manager to use judgment about other workers' competence when delegating responsibility to them. She is responsible not only for the care that the patients receive but also for how she has delegated care among the nursing staff (Mahlmeister 1999). She must balance the benefits of nursing care against the potential risks of not receiving care, without seriously jeopardising the health of any patient (Page 2004).

Any patient in the unit might be harmed by inadequate nursing staff levels. The ethical principles of beneficence, nonmaleficence and justice support nursing actions that maintain the trust between nurse and patient and that attempt to do good for patients without putting them at risk of preventable harm. These principles justify Ms Osako's actions. However, she seems to have little say about how long this situation may persist and what additional nursing resources might become available to her. A principle of justice would not support moving the elderly woman from the critical care unit to another unit if the level of care could not be guaranteed and if the patient's health would likely suffer as a result of the move. Under the circumstances, however, there seems little that Ms Osako can do other than protest about moving the new patient to the unit. This action seems unlikely, given her culture and her limited authority for managerial decisions.

What should be done?

To be an expert manager, Ms Osako must maintain a positive attitude toward her nursing staff; future patient care might suffer if nursing staff choose not to comply with management decisions. She is responsible to her co-workers for the way in which she manages their nursing skills and delegates authority to provide nursing care to patients. Although many nurse managers of critical care units throughout the world often receive advanced training and education for this role, they often do not have authority equal to their level of practice nor are they duly recognised for their ability to make complex decisions in the healthcare system.

One reason for the lack of nursing authority and recognition is the status and image of professional nursing. Despite the status of nursing as a profession having improved over the past several decades, in many parts of the world today nursing practice still has lower status than medical practice (Gordon 2005; Johnstone 1994; Perron & Holmes 2006; Thupayagale & Dithole 2005). The ability to be a competent and effective professional responsible for the delivery of therapeutically effective nursing care to patients will have little effect on patient care if others in the healthcare system, and the public, do not view the nurse as being a capable and competent professional who has a direct effect on patient outcomes (Gordon 2005; Page 2004). If nurses are to have a positive influence on how healthcare is delivered, then, regardless of the sociocultural contexts in which they are operating, they need to develop more assertive behaviours in clinical contexts and to become more politically involved and strategic generally in progressing processes aimed at improving the safety and quality of patient care as well as public health (Des Jardin 2001; Gordon 2005; Mahat & Phiri 1991). Ms Osako's values conflicts might be eased if her status as a nurse manager were changed and she was helped to become more assertive in her role. These changes will not help her in this situation but might prevent similar situations from occurring in the future. To change nursing's status and image and to increase nursing's authority, nurse managers need to work closely with their professional organisation to advance the practice of nursing in their countries and to gain more authority for nursing judgments and the planning of patient care (Gordon 2005; Johnstone 1994).

Accepting responsibility for nursing care

Nurses accept responsibility for nursing care in light of their nursing knowledge, competence, education and practice experience. If a nurse concludes that she is not adequately prepared or lacks competence to carry out expected functions, the nurse is responsible for notifying the nursing supervisor and refusing the assignment. Concern for patient safety and welfare prohibits nurses from accepting assignments that prevent them from fulfilling their ethical responsibilities to patients. The following case example demonstrates how ethical questions can arise about accepting responsibility for nursing care.

Exercise:

Case example 25: The nurse transferred to cover another unit[3]

What is the story behind the value conflicts?

Jean Wright is a licensed practical nurse (i.e. a second level nurse) who generally works the evening shift in a paediatric unit. Shortly after reporting to work, she is asked by the nursing supervisor to go to the maternity unit for a few hours. The registered nurse (RN) from the emergency room has had car trouble on the way to work and will be about two hours late. Since an RN is needed in the emergency room at all times, the supervisor is asking the maternity nurse to cover the emergency room until the other nurse arrives. The maternity floor is quiet and there is only one patient in early labour. Another nurse takes over Ms Wright's paediatric patients and she quickly goes to the maternity floor.

After an hour, the woman in labour begins to complain of a severe headache. Ms Wright checks the woman's vital signs and the fetal heart rate. The patient's blood pressure is 190/118, pulse 98, and respiration 24. The fetal heart rate is 156 and faint. The patient is becoming progressively restless and confused. Ms Wright calls the supervisor who is in the emergency room and asks her to send the other nurse back as she does not want to take responsibility for this patient. She does not feel competent to handle the situation and believes a physician should be called immediately. The supervisor promises to call a physician but says she cannot send back the RN to the maternity floor just yet. Several new admissions to the emergency room require the RN and the supervisor to remain there since the regular emergency room nurse has still not arrived. She urges Ms Wright to just keep taking the patient's vital signs and hang on. Ms Wright wonders why she agreed to be transferred to the maternity unit. If the condition of the labouring patient or her unborn infant deteriorates, is she responsible? Or does the supervisor bear all the responsibility?

Discussion questions

What is the significance of the values involved?

    (1)   Which values about patient care does Ms Wright seem to have?

(2) Which values about patient care are being expressed by the nursing supervisor?

(3) What values do we presume a pregnant patient to have about her care and that of her unborn infant?

(4) Are there any professional standards that might guide Ms Wright in accepting this responsibility for patient care?

(5) What are the responsibilities of any nurse who accepts care under the conditions in this case?

What is the significance of the conflicts to the parties involved?

(6) Which values appear to be in conflict with one another? Are the value conflicts significant for nursing practice? For the patient's health?

(7) How are the conflicts of values affecting Ms Wright's nursing practice? The nursing care of the patient?

(8) What are the options open to Ms Wright in this situation?

(9) What are the likely outcomes of each option? How might these outcomes affect Ms Wright? The woman and her infant?

(10) What does the discipline of ethics seem to offer to guide Ms Wright's actions?

What should be done?

(11) Which of the available options open to Ms Wright can be morally justified? Why?

(12) Which of the options cannot be morally justified? Why?

(13) If you were Ms Wright, what would you do in this situation? Why?

(14) What can you learn from this case situation about accepting responsibility for your nursing practice?

Summary

Most nurses learn to be competent practitioners of nursing from educational programmes. They learn basic theoretical knowledge that can be applied to many patient care situations. They learn clinical skills to carry out nursing measures and plan patient care. Nursing education does not protect them, however, from uncomfortable situations where they are called upon to allocate nursing resources, delegate nursing activities to others and be expected to give safe and competent nursing care in unfamiliar situations. Every nurse bears primary responsibility for his or her level of practice, for the safety of nursing interventions and for supervising others in giving nursing care.

In many situations, circumstances impede the competent, safe practice of nursing. When personnel are in short supply, supplies are inadequate, or care is being delivered in unsuitable environments, it is impossible to maintain the highest level of nursing care. Yet nurses are responsible for the care they provide under these less-than-ideal conditions. Increased nursing authority to deliver safe, competent and ethical nursing care will help ease some of these situations (Johnstone 1994). Changing the images of nurses, their knowledge and capabilities, will help change the expectations of nursing care and allow individual nurses to be more assertive in initiating and implementing ethical patient care (Gordon 2005). The ultimate goal is to provide the best possible care for the patient in a way that will improve people's health and well-being and reflect credit upon the nursing profession.

Notes

1 Adapted from Fry, S.T. & Veatch, R.M. (2006) *Case studies in nursing ethics*, 3rd ed. Boston: Jones & Bartlett Publishers (pp. 16–17). Used with permission.
2 Adapted from Fry, S.T. & Veatch, R.M. (2006) *Case studies in nursing ethics*, 3rd ed. Boston: Jones & Bartlett Publishers (p. 51). Used with permission.
3 Adapted from Fry, S.T. & Veatch, R.M. (2006) *Case studies in nursing ethics*, 3rd ed. Boston: Jones & Bartlett Publishers (pp. 45–46). Used with permission.

References

Aiken, L., Clarke, S., Cheung, R., Sloane, D. & Silber, J. (2003) Educational levels of hospital nurses and surgical patient mortality. *JAMA* 290(12), 1617–1623.

Beauchamp, T & Childress J. (2001) *Principles of biomedical ethics*, 5th ed. New York: Oxford University Press.

Christensen, C., Bohmer, R. & Kenagy, J. (2000) Will disruptive innovations cure health care? *Harvard Business Review* Sept–Oct, 102–112.

Daniels, N (2006) Equity and population health. *Hasts Ctr Rprt* 36(4), 22–35.

Des Jardin, K. (2001) Political involvement in nursing – politics, ethics, and strategic action. *AORN Journal* 74(5), 614–618.

Fry, S.T. & Veatch, R.M. (2006) *Case studies in nursing ethics*, 3rd ed. Boston: Jones & Bartlett Publishers.

Gordon, S. (2005) *Nursing against the odds: How health care cost cutting, media stereotyping, and medical hubris undermine nurses and patient care.* Ithaca & London: ILR Press, an imprint of Cornell University Press.

International Council of Nurses (ICN) (2000a) *Position statement: Management of nursing and health care services.* Geneva, Switzerland: ICN.

International Council of Nurses (ICN) (2000b) *Position statement: Assistive or support nursing personnel.* Geneva, Switzerland: ICN

International Council of Nurses (ICN) (2006) *Code of ethics for nurses.* Geneva, Switzerland: ICN.

Johnstone, M.-J. (1994) *Nursing and the injustices of the law.* Sydney: WB Saunders/ Baillière Tindall.

Johnstone, M.-J. (2004) *Bioethics: A nursing perspective*, 4th ed. Sydney: Elsevier/ Churchill Livingstone.

Kilner, J.T. (1995a) Macroallocation. In W.T. Reich (Ed) *Encyclopedia of bioethics*, 2nd ed (pp. 14331–14440). New York: Macmillan.

Kilner, J.F. (1995b) Microallocation. In W.T. Reich (Ed) *Encyclopedia of bioethics*, 2nd ed (pp. 14441–14542). New York: Macmillan.

Kurtzman, E. & Kizer, K. (2005) Evaluating the performance and contribution of nurses to achieve an environment of safety. *Nurs Admin Q* 29(1), 14–23.

Mahlmeister, L. (1999) Professional accountability and legal liability for the team leader and charge nurse. *JOGNN* 28(3), 300–309.

Mahat, G. & Phiri, M. (1991) Promoting assertive behaviors in traditional societies. *Intl Nurs Rev* 38(5), 153–155, 152.

Mucha, K. Fustos, M., Hoschke, E., Keszler, T., Kiss, L., Reisz, E. & Szabo, I. (1991) Developing nurse managers in Hungary. *Intl Nurs Rev* 38(5), 147–149.

Needleman, J., Buerhaus, P., Mattke, S., Stewart, M. & Zelevinsky, K. (2002) Nurse-staffing levels and the quality of care in hospitals. *NEJM* 346(22), 1715–1722.

Page, A. (Ed) (2004) *Keeping patients safe: Transforming the work environment of nurses.* Washington DC: National Academy Press.

Perron, A. & Holmes, D. (2006) Advanced practice: A clinical or political issue? *The Canadian Nurse* 102(7), 26–35.

Powers, M. & Faden, R. (2006) *Social justice: The moral foundations of public health and health policy.* New York: Oxford University Press.

Thupayagale, G. & Dithole, K. (2005) What is in a name: The case of nursing. *Nursing Forum* 40(4), 141–144.

Chapter 12
Nurses and the profession

Only individuals who have the knowledge, skills and commitment to practise nursing in a clinically, culturally and ethically competent manner should be admitted into the profession. This means that all nurses must be concerned about standards of nursing and how the competence of the nurse is achieved, measured, monitored, regulated and sustained (ICN 2003a, 2003b, 2005; Page 2004).

Nurse educators have a primary responsibility for ensuring the quality of nursing education and for ensuring that graduates of nursing programmes (whether undergraduate, postregistration, or postgraduate) achieve the competency standards (whether beginning or advanced) expected of them as licensed professionals. Practising nurses, on the other hand, are responsible for maintaining their competence once they are licensed. Nurse managers and administrators also share responsibility for ensuring that nurses are appropriately credentialed and competent to work in the areas to which they have been designated to work (Institute of Medicine 2001; Page 2004).

Maintaining one's competence to practice nursing requires continuing education throughout one's career, and sharing one's own knowledge and experience with colleagues. Through continuing education, research and scholarly inquiry, every nurse can contribute to the development of nursing knowledge and to nursing generally both as a profession and as a discipline. The nurse can be an educator, a researcher, an administrator, a manager, or a practitioner who tests theoretical foundations for practice and/or who uses tried and tested nursing measures pertinent to the delivery of safe and high quality patient care (ICN 2001, 2003a, 2003b).

Practising nurses are also responsible for working within an employer organisation to promote the value and cost-effectiveness of nursing as well as the socioeconomic welfare of nurses (ICN 2001, 2004a). Fulfilling this responsibility may include working cooperatively with others to establish and maintain equitable social and economic working conditions of nurses (ICN 2001, 2004a, 2004b, 2004c). To these ends, nurses collaborates with co-workers in bringing to the attention of employers and the members of the community their social and economic concerns, and other conditions that may pose barriers to achieving moral excellence in nursing (ICN 2001, 2004a, 2004b, 2004c; Johnstone 2001). In some instances, the nurse may, as a last resort, even need to participate in 'whistle blowing' or organised labour demonstrations to improve the social or economic conditions of nursing practice and, related to this, the capacity of nurses to provide moral care (ICN 2004a, 2004b, 2004c; Johnstone 1999, 2001, 2004a).

The International Council of Nurses (ICN) *Code of Ethics for Nurses* supports these functions of the nurse by stating that 'the nurse assumes the major role in determining and implementing acceptable standards of clinical nursing practice, management, research, and education' (2006, p. 3). It also notes that 'the nurse is active in developing a core of research-based professional knowledge', and 'acting through the professional organization, [the nurse] participates in creating and maintaining safe, equitable social and economic working conditions in nursing' (p. 3).

In this chapter, ethical conflicts experienced by nurses in trying to enhance the profession are explored. As this discussion indicates, the ethical concepts of advocacy, accountability, responsibility, cooperation and caring are very important to the values related to professional standards and education, nursing research and to the social and economic conditions of nursing.

Implementing desirable standards of nursing practice and nursing education

Implementing desired standards of nursing practice can be very difficult. First, nurses must agree on the standards. Second, nurses must be informed about the standards and the methods of evaluation used to determine whether a particular nurse is maintaining the standards in his or her practice. Third, nurses must be in an enabling environment, that is, in an environment that is supportive of the standards that nurses have agreed on and which they are expected to uphold (Johnstone 2001, 2004a; Page 2004). The following case situation demonstrates the questions one nurse had when the basis of accountability standards for his practice was not very clear.

Case example 26: How is nursing accountability determined?

What is the story behind the value conflicts?

George Steiner's job description for his new nursing position (Staff Nurse II) indicates that he is accountable for 'a high level of nursing competence and ethical nursing practice'. He asks his nursing supervisor how his job performance will be evaluated, especially where accountability for taking nursing responsibility is concerned. He learns that a panel of his peers will evaluate his nursing judgments in a variety of circumstances and patient care assignments. He will need to provide reasons for accepting specific patient care assignments and for his judgments in planning the care of those patients. Review of nurse accountability is highly recommended by his national nurses' association and his employer tries to implement the association's recommendations.

Mr Steiner is not a member of the national nurses' association and has no interest in their activities. He was not aware that nursing accountability in his place of employment is based on peer evaluations. He does not know if there are any external standards that he should be following in making nursing judgments, or whether his educational level is related to the nursing care assignments that he accepts. Why does he not know about accountability review? Should he try to delay his performance evaluation?

What is the significance of the values involved?

Mr Steiner has not previously valued his professional organisation. He has had no interest in the organisation and/or its activities. As a result, he is unaware of the organisation's efforts to set standards for nursing practice in his country and its recommendations for evaluating nursing competence and accountability. Perhaps his government does not encourage nurses to participate in a professional organisation. Perhaps his previous employer set its own standards for nursing practice and Mr Steiner thought it was only important to know and practise by those standards. Now, however, Mr Steiner is employed in a healthcare facility that sets standards for nursing practice according to those valued and promoted by the professional organisation. While it can be assumed that Mr Steiner values practising nursing in a clinically, culturally, ethically and legally safe and competent manner, he apparently does not value knowing the standards for these aspects of nursing practice; however, each nurse has a responsibility to know as well as to practise by these standards.

What is the significance of the conflicts to the parties involved?

Support of professional activities to implement higher standards for nursing practice is necessary. This support must come from several sources: legislation, the professional organisation, facilities that employ nurses and individual members of the profession. Nurses can be more effective in healthcare delivery if they have the support of their professional organisation. Nursing education can be more effective if the standards of nursing practice are accepted by the health ministry of the country and required of every nurse. Accepting, implementing and evaluating standards of nursing practice thus become the responsibility of every nurse.

What should be done?

By participating in their professional organisation, nurses become knowledgeable about the changing standards of nursing practice and how the nurse meets them. Mr Steiner needs to reconsider how valuable his professional organisation is to his career and how he can have a greater voice in determining the way he and his colleagues will be evaluated for their accountability. He needs to know more about external standards for nursing practice (including codes of ethics, codes of conduct, and related competency standards expected of licensed nurses), such as those supported and ratified by the professional organisation. He also needs to know what his responsibilities are according to his educational level in nursing. Many nursing organisations have developed position statements about areas of advanced nursing practice and the minimal educational levels required for and the competency standards expected of those working in these areas.

Mr Steiner also needs to learn more about how other nurses keep abreast of new developments in technology and nursing practice. Most professional nursing organisations support continuing education for nurses and help organise various seminars, conferences and other educational programmes. Participation in these activities will help every nurse to be better informed about employers' expectations and how the nurse's competence as well as professional (and moral) accountability is being assessed and evaluated.

Participating in research involving human participants

Nurses can also contribute to the development of the profession by conducting and participating in research involving human participants (ICN 1999) (Figure 12.1). Nurses can study nursing interventions and practices to make sure that they benefit patients and enhance their recovery from illness. They can also participate in research efforts by other members of the healthcare team so that the overall quality of patient care can be improved. Improved systems for the delivery of patient care, enhanced quality of nursing care and the implementation of nursing interventions that have been proven to be effective are all ways to influence the general health of society.

Research involving human participants often raises ethical issues, however. How much information needs to be given to a patient/participant in order for him or her to be properly informed about whether to participate in a given research project? Can a patient's participation in a research study be considered voluntary when the proposed nursing cares and treatments are available only under research conditions? How does the nurse researcher adequately assess the risks and benefits of an experimental treatment regimen? At what point will benefits

---

Position statement – Nursing research
Nursing research is needed to generate new knowledge, evaluate existing practice and services and provide evidence that will inform nursing education, practice, research and management.

- Research is directed toward understanding the fundamental mechanisms that affect the ability of individuals, families and communities to maintain or enhance optimum function and minimise the negative effects of illness.
- Nursing research should also be directed toward the outcomes of nursing interventions to assure the quality and cost effectiveness of nursing care.
- Nursing research also encourages:
  - knowledge of policies and systems that effectively and efficiently deliver nursing care,
  - awareness of the profession and its historical development,
  - understanding of ethical guidelines for the delivery of the nursing services,
  - knowledge of systems that effectively prepare nurses to fulfil the profession's current and future social mandate.

Figure 12.1   Excerpts from the ICN Position Statement (ICN 1999).

of a treatment under study become so apparent that the treatment should be offered to all patients in the study? Who will make this particular decision, the researcher or the prospective participant? Who decides ultimately what constitutes a benefit or risk and how great each respectively might be? These are questions that frequently confront nurse researchers and nurses in clinical practice when caring for patients and their families or chosen caregivers who have agreed to participate in a research study.

Ethical principles relevant to clinical research

The ethical principles discussed in Chapter 2 are all relevant to clinical research involving human participants. For example, the principle of autonomy applied to research means that research participants should be treated with respect and as having the capacity to make self-determining choices (Beauchamp & Childress 2001; Faden & Beauchamp 1986; NHMRC 2007). It also means that persons who are vulnerable, especially those with diminished capacity to make informed and self-determining choices in a research context, should be protected (Liamputtong 2006; Macklin 2003; Ruof 2004; Williams 2002).

Most national guidelines on human research ethics require that patients be given all relevant information about the research study that they have been approached about and in which they have been invited to participate. The kind of information that researchers are generally required to give to participants includes: details of who is conducting the research and why it is being conducted, what the project is about and the questions being addressed, why the participant has been approached and invited to participate, what he or she will be required to do if agreeing to and consenting to participate, what the possible risks and disadvantages are of participating, what the possible benefits are, what will happen with the information the participant provides, what rights the participant has (including the right to withdraw from the project at any time without prejudice; the right to have unprocessed data withdrawn and destroyed; the right to ask questions at any time), and whom to contact if requiring further information or if wishing to make a complaint (NHMRC 2001).

When participants are patients, they must also be told of the possible implications to their health and care of participating in the research project, including being reassured that if they choose not to participate or choose to withdraw after initially agreeing to participate, their care will not be compromised in any way. When age (e.g. the very young and the very old), illness, mental disability or other conditions restrict a patient's capacity to be self-determining, the nurse has a responsibility to take action to protect that patient from research activities that might otherwise disadvantage or harm them in some way (Kottow 2003; Macklin 2003; Ruof 2004; Williams 2002). Examples can include research activities that compromise the patient's safety and quality of care, their health, their privacy, dignity and so forth.

The principles of beneficence and nonmaleficence applied to research mean that researchers have an obligation to maximise possible benefits and to minimise possible harms that might occur in a research context (Fry & Veatch 2006). This is a difficult task as sometimes it is impossible to know for certain what is beneficial and what is harmful unless it is tested. Sometimes it is justified to seek some benefits even though risks are involved. At other times, benefiting the patient through research should not even be attempted because of significant risks to the patient. Researchers must present all the known information about risks and benefits to the patient since it is only the patient and/or guardian who can make an authentic decision to accept or reject the possible risks and benefits that are associated with a given project.

The principle of justice applied to research means that the researcher must select research participants carefully to avoid taking advantage of or disadvantaging vulnerable people (Liamputtong 2006; Macklin 2003; Rouf 2004; Williams 2002). The research project design also may create questions about fairness to research participants and the manner in which benefits and risks are assigned to them.

Ethical issues in clinical research

Three major ethical issues in clinical research are:

(1) informed consent
(2) determination of benefit-to-risk ratios
(3) privacy and confidentiality

Informed consent

Before a research project commences, the consent of participants must be obtained unless there are special and carefully defined circumstances, such as those specified in a national human research ethics guideline (e.g. see NHMRC 2007; Spriggs 2004), that may enable consent to be waived. The requirement to obtain consent has two key dimensions: (i) the provision of information, and (ii) the capacity to decide and to make a voluntary choice to participate.

The principle of autonomy requires that research participants be given 'the opportunity to choose what shall or shall not happen to them' (Beauchamp & Childress 2001). They are given this opportunity when adequate provisions for informed consent are included in the research protocol. Informed consent is a process that protects research participants' autonomy, protects participants from harm, and helps the researcher to avoid fraud and duress in healthcare and associated research contexts. It also encourages professional responsibility for how information is communicated in research contexts, promotes reasoned decision making by the participant, and involves the public in promoting self-determination as a social value.

Informed consent has three essential components: information, voluntariness, and competence (Faden & Beauchamp 1986; NHMRC 2007). All three of these components must be evident for a participant's consent to be truly informed.

Information

For adequate disclosure of information, the research participant must be informed of the procedures to be used throughout the study (Fry & Veatch 2006). Information about available alternative treatment procedures, a discussion of risks and benefits of these procedures and the opportunity for questions about or withdrawal from the project after treatment has begun, should all be provided to the research participant.

For adequate comprehension of information, the research participant must have time to consider the information and to ask questions. This means that when the ability to comprehend information is limited (for example, when the patient's mental competence is limited), the researcher needs to allow the research participant additional opportunity to consider whether or not to participate in the study.

Voluntariness

'Voluntary consent' to participate in research means that the participant has exercised his or her choice free of coercion and other forms of controlling influence by other persons. A research participant's consent is only valid if it is given voluntarily (Fry & Veatch 2006). Voluntariness protects the patient's right to choose his or her own goals and to choose among several goals when offered options.

Competence

People ('mature minors' as well as adults) are generally considered to competent and able to give consent if they can demonstrate that they have the capacity to appreciate the nature, risks and consequences of a procedure (Derish & Vanden Heuvel 2000). It is acknowledged that competence may be difficult to assess (Grisso & Appelbaum 1998; Johnstone 2004b; NHMRC 2007). Nonetheless, in research contexts, informed consent to participate cannot be given unless the patient or research participant is 'competent' to decide, that is, has the capacity to appreciate the nature, risks and consequences of participating in the research at hand.

Determination of benefit-to-risk ratios

Determining benefit and risk ratios is one of the more difficult problems that a researcher may encounter during the planning and carrying out of a research protocol (see, for example, Allmark et al. 2001; Clark 2002). The researcher must consider all possible consequences of the research design and be willing to balance any inherent risks to the research participant with proportionate benefit to that person. This includes identifying those persons most likely to be subject to risk in the study, identifying the types and level of risk involved (physical, psychological/emotional, cultural and social) and identifying (also quantifying) the anticipated benefits to the participants in the research study (Allmark et al. 2001; Clark 2002; Hirshon et al. 2002; Johnstone 2007). Only by identifying all of these factors can a satisfactory determination of the benefit-to-risk ratio be made and process put in place to ensure the protection of participants should an anticipated risk become realised. Without a determination of the benefit-to-risk ratio, moral justification of the research study will always remain in question. Failure to properly assess and anticipate the material risks of a proposed project may also make it vulnerable to legal consequence later should 'something go wrong' (Mello et al. 2003).

Privacy and confidentiality

Privacy is a complex notion that derives from a special moral interest that people have in 'having control over information about themselves' and about 'who else should have access to that information' – when, how and under what conditions (Johnstone 2004b, p. 162). Thus, the principle of privacy is primarily concerned with information and the conditions under which certain information that has been collected (in this instance, in a research context) is shared (NHMRC 2001).

This 'right to privacy' is linked in important ways to the moral principle of autonomy, which prescribes that people should be respected as self-determining choosers. Thus, if a person autonomously chooses to have certain information about themselves kept private or 'secret', provided this choice does not harm or prejudice the significant moral interests of others, this choice must be upheld (Johnstone 2004b, p. 162). Under human research ethics guidelines, researchers are generally reminded that they have both a legal and an ethical obligation not to use information gained in a research context 'for any purpose other than that for which it was given' and, moreover, that every reasonable effort will be made to protect (keep confidential) the identities of participants, such as by de-identifying the information collected (NHMRC 2007). This means that anyone associated with a given research project and coming into contact with personal information about a participant is obliged – morally and legally – to keep that information private.

The following case illustrates how ethical questions and the above ethical issues can arise in research studies designed to test the effectiveness of nursing measures in patient care.

Case example 27: Benefits and harms in a nursing research study[1]

What is the story behind the value conflicts?

Mrs Helga Koch is the nurse in charge of a cardiovascular nursing care unit. For the past two years, the nurses on the unit have been studying the physiological and psychological effects of self-care activities in patients recovering from myocardial infarctions. Patients admitted to the unit have been carefully screened and selected according to medical data such as:

(1) minimal amount of myocardial damage suffered
(2) absence of known cardiovascular disease prior to the present illness
(3) excellent prognosis of the patient

To date, a significant positive correlation between self-care activities and psychological status among the study patients has been found.

Mrs Koch and the other nurses would like to include other patients in the study such as those having more extensive myocardial damage and those with known cardiovascular disease prior to this hospital admission. Related studies have indicated that this type of patient has a higher incidence of depression and other psychological problems, as well as noncompliance in follow-up treatment. Mrs Koch and the other nurses want to find out whether early self-care activities in patient care affect the incidence of depression and other psychological problems and compliance to treatment in these patients.

The physician in charge of the unit has no objection to including these patients in the nurses' study. Yet Mrs Koch is uncertain whether it is ethical to do so. She knows that the use of self-care activities in planning nursing care for these patients poses some risks. But she does not know how serious these risks might be. Although she believes that the self-care activities will have a beneficial effect on the psychological status of these patients and may increase compliance to treatment, she is not certain that this will occur. Is it ethical for Mrs Koch to include these patients in the study?

What is the significance of the values involved?

The development, promotion and implementation of evidence-based nursing practice is critical to ensuring the delivery of safe and quality care to patients and to achieving 'good' patient outcomes (Courtney 2005). Evidence-based nursing practice is also critical to improving the credibility of the nursing profession and to enabling nurses to be both morally and legally accountable for their practice (Courtney 2005; Dawes et al. 2005; Page 2004). To achieve the goals of nursing research, however, research plans need to be developed and carried out in strict accordance with the ultimate standards of competent and ethical research. Research that is poorly designed or conducted in a sub-standard, unethical and even fraudulent manner not only risks exposing participants unnecessarily to the burdens of engaging in 'useless' research, but risks bringing the research community itself into disrepute (Fernandez 2005; McNeill 1993; NHMRC 2007). It can also result in otherwise avoidable harm being caused to participants.

The nursing profession has an interest in, and values being able to demonstrate by way of valid and credible research, evidence of good nursing care. Patients and their families or chosen caregivers also have an interest in receiving good nursing care based on research evidence rather than nursing care based on tradition. Evidence-based practice is the hallmark of an accountable and responsible profession.

What is the significance of the conflicts to the parties involved?

No research is risk free. All researchers (including nurse researchers) and those who assist them have a stringent moral responsibility to ensure that the welfare and rights of participants in research are protected, and that every reasonable measure is taken to prevent harm or at least minimise the risk of harm being caused to them during all phases of a research project, i.e. from the recruitment of prospective participants through to the dissemination of a study's findings. Such measures must include the honest and ethical design and conduct of the research as well as the dissemination and communication of its results, careful screening of prospective participants in strict accordance with inclusion criteria which have been carefully and competently devised, the ethical recruitment of participants, a rigorous and independent assessment of risks associated with the proposed research, identification of readily accessible support mechanisms if harm should occur, and ready access to the institutional research or ethics committee responsible for approving the research plan should advice be required or should a participant wish to make a complaint. When assessing risk, careful attention must be given to identifying the particular risks of harm that may arise in a proposed study, assessing the magnitude of each of the risks identified and the probability of each of the risks identified occurring, and the processes a researcher has put in place to minimise both the incidence and possible impact of the risks identified become a reality (NHMRC 2007).

What should be done?

To include the new category of patients (e.g. those whose conditions are more serious) would raise practical questions about research protocol and design. The nurse researchers wishing to include this new category of patients need to submit another research proposal for approval by the institutional research or ethics committee. The proposal needs to define clearly the inclusion criteria for the expanded study they are proposing, a comprehensive and exhaustive assessment of the risk or benefits of including the more seriously ill category of patients, processes for reducing participant vulnerability and strategies for minimising the known and reasonably anticipated risks associated with including the more seriously ill class of patients. Mrs Koch should discuss this with the nurse research team. If the nurse researchers do not agree to submit a new research plan to the institutional research or ethics committee to obtain approval for expanding the scope of their original study, that is, to include the new category of patients, it would be appropriate for Mrs Koch to approach the institutional research or ethics committee directly to have the matter resolved.

Equitable social and economic working conditions in nursing

In many countries, nurses join labour unions as a means of bargaining for better working conditions. The labour union may or may not promote the same standards of nursing practice established by the professional organisation. The following case example describes how nurses can experience ethical conflict after participating in an organised labour dispute to achieve job security.

Case example 28: Striking as a means to protest clinical grading

What is the story behind the value conflicts?

Joanna T participated in a strike with 120 other nurses because two nurses at Joanna's institution were suspended following a dispute over clinical grading and job promotion. Nurses at two other hospitals in the region participated in the strike and all nurses were members of labour unions. The nurses at each hospital arranged for emergency staffing of nursing units during the two-week strike. Now, 18 months later, Joanna and the majority of the nurses who took part in the strike are being investigated for alleged professional misconduct. It seems that several anonymous complaints about the care of patients during the strike have been forwarded to the investigative board.

Is participating in a strike the same as abandoning one's patients? Is participating in a strike unethical behaviour on the part of the nurse?

What is the significance of the values involved?

Joanna T and the other nurses who participated in this organised strike apparently value nursing control of judgments related to clinical grading. Their decision to strike is made on behalf of two other nurses who have been economically harmed by being suspended from their jobs. Disagreement with employers and seeking redress for the employer's clinical evaluation of nursing status are not cause for suspension or dismissal. The nurses value job security and cooperation among nurses in ensuring economic safeguards within the nurse workforce. The nurses do not, however, have much respect for the professional organisation's ability to address labour disputes which is why they have joined labour unions.[2]

The nurses value the health and well-being of their patients as demonstrated by the emergency care provided to patients during the two-week strike. Moreover, the 'skeleton' nursing workforce providing nursing services during the strike is appropriately qualified and competent to provide safe and prudent care. Ironically, because the hospital's operations have been reduced in response to the strike, nurse–patient ratios are better than usual – even with the majority of nursing staff being on strike leave.

The employing hospitals, on the other hand, value management's oversight and control of nursing practice, wage setting and employment security. The hospitals believe that they can hire the nurses they want and dismiss them without notice if the nurses complain or question management's decisions. Since nursing practice is still under the control of medicine or considered not to be a profession in many parts of the world, or is under the control of business managers who have little appreciation of the value and cost-effectiveness of competent nursing care, many nurses have little opportunity to speak out on issues of economic and job security. For nurses in many countries (including those which have highly developed and well-resourced healthcare services), joining a labour union may be the only way they can address these issues. In some countries, however, professional nursing organisations are also concerned about such issues and are beginning to work effectively with nurses to address them. Nurses need to consider whether they can best address social and economic issues through labour disputes or by raising the standards of professional nursing through active participation in education, legislative reform, political lobbying, policy development and organisational influence (Des Jardin 2001; Gordon 2005; ICN 2000a, 2000b).

What is the significance of the conflicts to the parties involved?

Nurses are obligated to assist their professional organisation in establishing equitable social and economic conditions in nursing. Joanna T and her colleagues certainly agree that they have a right to the same job security as physicians and other health workers. However, each nurse probably supports herself or contributes to the support of a family and does not want to do anything to jeopardise her position, steady income and support for self or family. By participating in labour disputes or even in the professional organisation's support of nursing strikes, they may be fired by employers or charged with professional misconduct, making it difficult for them to find a job somewhere else. This is the conflict that Joanna T and the other nurses face, months after participating in the labour dispute.

It seems that Joanna T and the nurses are being 'punished' for participating in the strike. If found guilty of abandoning patients during the strike – unethical and illegal actions on the part of the nurses – they may have their licences to practise revoked. While striking for the protection of patient safety and well-being is not considered unethical behaviour for nurses, many believe that striking to improve one's own job security is not ethical nursing behaviour.

What should be done?

The nurses charged with professional misconduct will have to show that striking for economic reasons is not unethical. They will need to establish that economic security promotes better patient care and guarantees that certain standards of nursing practice will be maintained in all of the hospitals. Less turnover in staff, a stronger commitment to the employing hospital, and increased nursing responsibility for patient care standards have all been shown to contribute to the quality of patient care, as perceived by patients (Aiken et al. 2001, 2003; Needleman et al. 2002; Page 2004). If the nurses can convince others that these are their ultimate goals in striking for job security, then they will have a stronger case (ICN 2004a, 2004b, 2004c; Johnstone 1999).

The nurses can document that the nurses retained during the strike were educationally prepared for their patient care responsibilities and were employed to protect patients from harm. They can also demonstrate that the professional organisation supports nurses' strikes on behalf of patient safety and improved outcomes as well as economic security of nurses.

In the following case example, nurses strike for a reason related more to the protection of nurses than to the protection of patients. Is striking for these reasons unethical?

Exercise:

Case example 29: Collective action for self-protection in providing nursing care

What is the story behind the value conflicts?

In a developed country with a well-developed and well-resourced healthcare system, 1100 members of a national nursing organisation walked off duty after weeks of negotiation had provided no solution to the nurses' demands. The nurses had asked for safe transportation to and from their employment sites in order to avoid personal assaults and sexual harassment, particularly when reporting for afternoon, night and weekend shifts. The strike provoked public condemnation of the employers for failure to consider the nurses' risks when reporting to work or returning to their homes. As a result of the incident, a review of the nursing profession and its duties has been recommended by the national government. Will these nurses' actions contribute to societal good? How will patient good be served through these events?

Discussion questions

What is the significance of the values?

(1) What values support the nurses' reasons for striking? Are these values moral or nonmoral in nature?
(2) What values are implied by the public outcry against the employers of nurses?
(3) Do these values have meaning for the citizens of the country? If so, in what way? If not, why not?
(4) Where do you think values conflicts exist for the employing hospitals? For the nurses? For citizens?

What is the significance of the conflicts to the parties involved?

(5) How might the care of future patients be affected by the values conflicts?
(6) What are the duties of nurses to safeguard patient safety and well-being? Are these duties to be performed at personal risk to the nurse? Why or why not?
(7) How have the conflicts likely affected nursing practice in this country? Do you perceive this as good or bad?
(8) How have the values conflicts led to policy formation?

What should be done?

(9) Should the review of nurses' duties be accomplished by non-nurses or nurses? Why?
(10) What role should the ethical duties of nurses have in situations of this nature?
(11) How do you think the conflicts between the nurses and the employers should have been handled before the walk-out?
(12) Was the walk-out unethical behaviour for professional nurses? Why or why not?
(13) How would you work toward promoting job safety in your employment setting? How would you support your judgments with ethical principles and concepts of nursing?

Summary

The ethical duties of nurses apply to all roles that they assume as educators, managers, administrators, researchers and clinical workers. When social or economic conditions constrain the ethical practice of nursing, the ethical duties of nurses must be balanced against the goals of organised labour disputes, strikes and nurse walk-outs (ICN 2004a, 2004b, 2004c; Johnstone 1999). Participation in the professional organisation is one way that nurses can find support for their efforts to raise standards of nursing practice and education, and to establish equitable social and economic conditions in nursing practice. Ultimately, all nurses play important roles in developing the knowledge base for nursing practice and for maintaining the professional and ethical standards against which nurses' conduct will be evaluated.

Notes

1   Adapted from Fry, S.T. & Veatch, R.M. (2006) *Case studies in nursing ethics*, 3rd ed. Boston, Jones & Bartlett Publishers (pp. 336–337). Used with permission.
2   In some countries, the professional nurses' organisation/association is a labour union or at least functions as a labour union. In other countries, professional nurses' associations and labour unions are separate organisations.

References

Aiken, L., Clarke, S., Sloane, D., Sochalski, J., Busse, R., Clarke, H., Giovannetti, P., Hunt, J., Rafferty, A. & Shamian, J. (2001) Nurses' reports on hospital care in five countries. *Health Affairs* 20(3), 43–53.

Aiken, L., Clarke, S., Cheung, R., Sloane, D. & Silber, J. (2003) Educational levels of hospital nurses and surgical patient mortality. *JAMA* 290(12), 1617–1623.

Allmark, P., Mason, S., Gill, A. & Megone, C. (2001) Is it in a neonate's best interest to enter a randomised controlled trial? *Journal of Medical Ethics* 27(2), 110–113.

Beauchamp, T. & Childress, J. (2001) *Principles of biomedical ethics*, 5th ed. New York: Oxford University Press.

Clark, P. (2002) Placebo surgery for Parkinson's disease: Do the benefits outweigh the risks? *Journal of Law, Medicine & Ethics* 30(1), 58–68.

Courtney, M. (Ed) (2005) *Evidence for nursing practice*. Sydney: Elsevier/Churchill Livingstone.

Dawes, M., Davies, P., Gray, A., Mant, J., Seers, K. & Snowball, R. (2005) *Evidence-based practice: A primer for health care professionals*. Edinburgh: Elsevier/Churchill Livingstone.

Derish, M. & Vanden Heuvel, K. (2000) Mature minors should have the right to refuse life-sustaining medical treatment. *Journal of Law, Medicine & Ethics* 28, 109–124.

Des Jardin, K. (2001) Political involvement in nursing – politics, ethics, and strategic action. *AORN Journal* 74(5), 614–618.

Faden, R. & Beauchamp, T.L. (1986) *A history and theory of informed consent*. New York: Oxford University Press.

Fernandez, C. (2005) Publication of ethically suspect research: Should it occur? *International Journal for Quality in Health Care* 17(5), 377–378.

Fry, S.T. & Veatch, R.M. (2006) *Case studies in nursing ethics*, 3rd ed. Boston: Jones & Bartlett Publishers.

Gordon, S. (2005) *Nursing against the odds: How health care cost cutting, media stereotyping, and medical hubris undermine nurses and patient care*. Ithaca & London: ILR Press, an imprint of Cornell University Press.

Grisso, T. & Appelbaum, P. (1998) *Assessing competence to consent to treatment: A guide for physicians and other health professionals*. New York: Oxford University Press.

Hirshon, J., Krugman, S., Witting, M., Furuno, J., Limcangco, M., Perisse, A. & Rasch, E. (2002) Variability in institutional review board assessment of minimal-risk research. *Acad Emerg. Med* 9(12), 1417–1420.

Institute of Medicine (2001) *Crossing the quality chasm: A new health system for the 21st Century*. Washington, DC: National Academy Press.

International Council of Nurses (ICN) (1999) *Position statement: Nursing research.* Geneva: ICN.

International Council of Nurses (ICN) (2000a) *Position statement: Management of nursing and health care services.* Geneva: ICN.

International Council of Nurses (ICN) (2000b) *Position statement: Participation of nurses in health services decision making and policy development.* Geneva: ICN.

International Council of Nurses (ICN) (2001) *Position statement: Promoting the value and cost-effectiveness of nursing.* Geneva: ICN.

International Council of Nurses (ICN) (2003a) *ICN Framework of competencies for the generalist nurse.* Geneva: ICN.

International Council of Nurses (ICN) (2003b) *An implementation model for the ICN framework of competencies for the generalist nurse.* Geneva: ICN.

International Council of Nurses (ICN) (2004a) *Position statement: Socio-economic welfare of nurses.* Geneva: ICN.

International Council of Nurses (ICN) (2004b) *Position statement: Strike policy.* Geneva: ICN

International Council of Nurses (ICN) (2004c) *Guidelines on essential services during labour conflict.* Geneva: ICN.

International Council of Nurses (ICN) (2005) *Nursing regulation: A futures perspective.* Geneva: ICN.

International Council of Nurses (ICN) (2006) *Code of ethics for nurses.* Geneva: ICN.

Johnstone, M.-J. (1999) Strike action. In M. Johnstone (Ed) *Bioethics: A nursing perspective*, 3rd ed (pp. 407–416). Sydney: Harcourt/Saunders.

Johnstone, M.-J. (2001) Poor working conditions and the capacity of nurses to provide moral care. *Contemporary Nurse* 12(1), 7–15.

Johnstone, M.-J. (2004a) Patient safety, ethics and whistleblowing: A nursing response to the events at the Campbelltown and Camden Hospitals. *Australian Health Review* 28(1), 13–19.

Johnstone, M.-J. (2004b) *Bioethics: a nursing perspective*, 4th ed. Sydney: Elsevier/ Churchill Livingstone.

Johnstone, M.-J. (2007) Research ethics, reconciliation, and strengthening the research relationship in indigenous health domains: An Australian perspective. *International Journal of Intercultural Relations* 31(3), 391–406.

Kottow, M. (2003) The vulnerable and the susceptible. *Bioethics* 17(5–6), 460–471.

Liamputtong, P. (2006) *Researching the vulnerable: A guide to sensitive research methods.* London, UK: Sage Publications.

Macklin, R. (2003) Bioethics, vulnerability, and protection. *Bioethics* 17(5–6), 472–486.

McNeill, P. (1993) *The ethics and politics of human experimentation.* Cambridge, UK: Cambridge University Press.

Mello, M., Studdert, D. & Brennan, T. (2003) The rise of litigation in human subjects research. *Annals of Internal Medicine* 139(1), 40–45.

National Health & Medical Research Council (NHMRC) (2007) *National statement on ethical conduct in human research.* Canberra: NHMRC.

Needleman, J., Buerhaus, P., Mattke, S., Stewart, M. & Zelevinsky, K. (2002) Nurse-staffing levels and the quality of care in hospitals. *NEJM* 346(22), 1715–1722.

Page, A. (Ed) (2004) *Keeping patients safe: Transforming the work environment of nurses.* Washington DC: National Academy Press.

Ruof, M. (2004) Scope notes 44: Vulnerability, vulnerable populations, and policy. *KEIJ* 14(4), 411–425.

Spriggs, M. (2004) Canaries in the mines: Children, risk, non-therapeutic research, and justice. *Journal of Medical Ethics* 30(2), 176–181.

Williams, A. (2002) Issues of consent and data collection on vulnerable populations. *Journal of Neuroscience Nursing* 34(4), 211–217.

Chapter 13
Nurses and co-workers

The ethical concept of advocacy gives the nurse's role a very important dimension in patient care. As discussed in Chapter 3, the nurse has a responsibility to protect the patient whenever health and well-being are endangered by anyone else and is accountable to the patient, his or her family, the profession and even society for how the advocacy role is carried out. For example, the nurse protects the basic human values of the patient, such as self-determination, privacy and dignity. The nurse may even need to protect the patient from co-workers' actions that could endanger the patient and cause him or her significant moral harm.

Being a patient advocate gives the nurse a somewhat adversarial role in healthcare. The nurse at the bedside defends the patient and watches to make sure that the patient is protected from the harms of preventable adverse events. If anyone involved in the patient's care acts in an unsafe, unethical or incompetent manner, the nurse is expected to report this or 'takes appropriate action to safeguard individuals, families, and communities when their health is endangered by a co-worker or any other person' (International Council of Nurses (ICN) 2006, p. 3).

At the same time, the nurse is expected to establish and sustain 'a cooperative relationship with co-workers in nursing and other fields' (p. 3). This means that the nurse participates in collaborative planning with other healthcare workers at all administrative and regulatory levels of the healthcare system to enhance patient outcomes. It also means that nurses should strive for an interdisciplinary approach to the delivery of services. While many nurses do participate and collaborate with their co-workers, other nurses often experience lack of cooperation from co-workers, especially from physician colleagues. Why does this occur and how do uncooperative relationships with co-workers, especially physicians, create ethical conflicts in patient care?

Cooperating with physicians

Nurses tend to perceive their relationships with physicians differently from the way physicians perceive their relationships with nurses (Marrone 2003; Oberle & Hughes 2001). In years past, the nurse ideally described the nurse–physician relationship as collegial in nature (Davidhizar & Dowd 2003). It was described as a relationship that included mutual consideration and mutual sharing of information about the patient. Unfortunately, the majority of nurses in clinical practice do not experience this type of relationship with a physician. Physicians often view the nurse as an obedient and compliant individual who is primarily responsive to the physician and only secondarily responsive to the patient (Castledine 2004).

The physician's view of the nurse–patient relationship was popularised in the 1960s and called the Doctor/Nurse Game (Stein 1967). In the Game, the physician is superior to the nurse and their interactions are carefully managed so as not to disturb this hierarchy. Nurses can be bold and innovative in playing the Game but must seem passive while they are doing it. Nurses can make recommendations about patient care, but their recommendations must appear to be initiated by the physician (Stein 1967). Open disagreement between physician and nurse is avoided at all costs. If both physician and nurse play the Game successfully, the team operates efficiently and the nurse is considered the physician's consultant. This position gives the nurse self-esteem and the physician is generally admired by the nursing staff. If the Game is not played well, penalties occur on both sides. Physicians who fail to recognise the nurses' subtle recommendations in the approved manner are not respected. If they resent the nurses' suggestions, the nurses 'pay them back' by being uncooperative. If nurses are too outspoken, they are demeaned and treated as troublemakers. To play the Game well is the main objective. Quality of patient care is a secondary objective.

Fortunately, the 'rules of the Game' are changing between physicians and nurses. The image of the nurse as an obedient and compliant individual is slowly giving way to that of a specialist certified in advanced practice with independent duties and responsibilities to patients (Stein, Watts & Howell 1990). Many physicians now depend on nurses' expertise. Physicians more often view their collaborative relationships with other healthcare workers as equal partnerships (Ashworth 2000; Iacono 2003).

One reason for this change in physician–nurse relationships is advanced education for nurses. In the academic environment, students in the health professions are taught that nurses are professionals responsible for making decisions and are accountable for the results of those decisions. Nursing students are also being taught to communicate with physicians very differently from how they communicated in the past (Castledine 2004; Homsted 2003). This does not mean, however, that conflicts between physicians and nurses do not occur. Conflicts are common and often unavoidable, but how they are handled depends, in part, on how each professional views the relationship and the nature of the conflict (LeTourneau 2004; Tabak & Orit 2007).

Ethical conflicts between physicians and nurses over patient care are the most frequently experienced ethical problems described by nurses in clinical practice (Arndt 1999; Ashworth 2000). The following case example demonstrates one type of ethical conflict often experienced by nurses in their relationships with physicians.

Case example 30: How far should the nurse go in promoting a child's health?[1]

What is the story behind the value conflicts?

Mrs Chou, a school health nurse, recently referred an 8-year-old child to the clinic physician for a hearing assessment. The child's teacher had noticed that the child was having problems in his schoolwork and did not pay attention in the classroom. Mrs Chou examined the child physically and then referred him to a specialised clinic for a hearing assessment. The test results were then sent to the child's paediatrician with the recommendation that the child receive continued follow-up. Several months later, the nurse asked the teacher about the child's progress. She learned that the parents had been told the test results were normal and no cause for the poor schoolwork had been found. When the nurse called the paediatrician for further information, he indicated that the child did not need specialised education, and could continue in the regular school system. He told the nurse that she need not concern herself with the child's problems as he and the family were handling the situation. The nurse then requested a full report of the test results through the clinic. The report showed her initial assessment to be correct: the child had a marked bilateral hearing loss requiring a hearing aid and a special educational programme had been recommended to help the child catch up with his classmates. Should she call the unfriendly paediatrician again and persist in raising questions about this child's poor schoolwork and his follow-up?

What is the significance of the values involved?

Mrs Chou obviously wants to promote the health of the child with a hearing loss. She wants to prevent further loss of the child's hearing and provide for the special educational needs that resulted from the hearing loss. Carrying out this responsibility, however, places her in conflict with the child's paediatrician. She cannot adequately promote the health of the child and request special education without the assistance of the physician. Yet, in order to obtain his assistance, she must confront him about what she has learned from the report of the test results.

The physician values his judgment about the severity of the child's hearing deficit and his relationship with the family. He values his role as decision maker where promotion of the child's health is concerned. The physician does not seem to value Mrs. Chou's assessment of the child and her knowledge of the hearing test results.

What is the significance of the conflicts to the parties involved?

Some nurses might find the possibility of open disagreement with the physician so undesirable that they would avoid any confrontational discussions with him. They would accept his authority in the situation without question, despite the results of the hearing test. They would not concern themselves with the child's hearing 'problem' again, but assume that the physician and the parents were taking care of whatever follow-up they deemed necessary. The nurse–physician relationship would be preserved and the physician would regard the nurse as obedient. Unfortunately, this action by the nurse would not promote the health or education of the child.

One way to avoid direct confrontation with the paediatrician would be for Mrs Chou to share what she has learned with the parents and urge them to question the paediatrician. Though avoiding direct confrontation with the paediatrician, this course of action might damage the nurse–physician relationship as he will surely learn that the nurse has urged the parents to raise these questions. Working through the parents very likely will lessen their confidence in the paediatrician since they believe that the child's hearing is normal. If the overall goal is to promote the child's health, this does not seem to be a desirable outcome of the nurse's actions.

What should be done?

Promoting the child's health may require the nurse to act as an advocate and collaborator by working with the child's school and teacher, the clinic services and the child's paediatrician. In many areas of the world, school nurses are the first line of health promotion for the school-age child and are indispensable in the prevention of chronic disease among this population group. While it is important to maintain collegial relationships with co-workers, especially physicians, the nurse's primary responsibility to promote children's health carries great moral weight and takes precedence over all other responsibilities (ICN 2000). This means that Mrs Chou cannot avoid her moral responsibility to follow up on the care and educational placement of the child. Promoting this child's health will require her involvement with the teacher, the child's family and the paediatrician. She has a responsibility to discuss the situation openly with the physician and the child's parents. She must also see that the parents and the teacher confer so that suitable educational arrangements for the child can be arranged.

Cooperating with nurses and other co-workers

As discussed in Chapter 3, the ethical concept of cooperation is defined as active participation with others to obtain quality care for patients, collaboration in designing nursing care and reciprocity with other nurses. Cooperating with other nurses means working with them toward shared goals and giving priority to mutual concerns about patient care. It also means being willing to compromise on individual and/or personal values when doing so will preserve individual integrity and cooperative relationships (Fry 2004). It does not mean being blindly loyal to anything important simply because it was generated by nurses or because it relates to nursing care.

Ethical conflict can occur, however, whenever the nurse is uncertain about what or whose values are actually being promoted by cooperation between nurses. The following case situation demonstrates the ethical questions faced by one nurse when she was asked to cooperate with her nurse colleagues.

Case example 31: When no one likes the acting head nurse

What is the story behind the value conflicts?

Maria Sanchez has worked on a busy medical care unit since she graduated from nursing school two years ago. Several months ago, the head nurse, respected and liked by everyone, moved to another city. Another nurse, Mrs Montoya, was appointed Acting Head Nurse since she had worked on the unit longer than anyone else.

While she is a good bedside nurse, Mrs Montoya does not seem to have the managerial and political skills of the previous head nurse. Her mistakes in assigning patient care and scheduling the nurses' work have led to dissatisfaction among the nurses. When the nurses have asked her about their work schedules, Mrs Montoya has refused to make changes. She does not take criticism well, refuses to acknowledge her own mistakes and openly criticises some of the nurses, causing hurt and embarrassment. A few of the nurses have become quite resentful of this kind of treatment.

Miss Sanchez and the other nurses learn that Mrs Montoya is applying for the position of head nurse. Although she has not personally experienced any problems with Mrs Montoya, Miss Sanchez believes that Mrs Montoya is not a good head nurse. She is also concerned about the poor working relationships that have developed among the nurses since Mrs Montoya was appointed Acting Head Nurse. Mrs Montoya, however, is supported by the administration and the physicians. The other nurses on the unit ask Miss Sanchez to join them in communicating to the hospital administration their negative feelings about Mrs Montoya and their lack of support for her as head nurse. They plan to discuss their feelings directly with the resident physician and the Director of Nursing, and report their various dissatisfactions with Mrs Montoya. They will not tell Mrs Montoya of their intent to speak to the Director of Nursing because they do not believe that meeting with Mrs Montoya to air their dissatisfaction with her leadership will change anything. The nurses tell Miss Sanchez that it is important for all the staff nurses to 'stick together' and cooperate with one another in presenting their views about Mrs Montoya to the Director of Nursing and the resident physician. Is Miss Sanchez obligated to participate in these plans in the name of professional cooperation?

What is the significance of the values involved?

There seem to be different values being promoted in this case example. Mrs Montoya values bedside nursing care and the role of head nurse. It is important to her to be named to this position as the most senior nurse clinician on the unit. While she values the title that comes with the position, she does not especially value the quality of working relationships among the nursing staff and how her leadership (or lack thereof) affects the staff. Disgruntled staff nurses do not bother her as long as they do their work and the patients are adequately cared for.

The nurses, on the other hand, value respectful treatment, consideration of their own needs as well as patient needs and satisfying working conditions. They also value cooperation as a means to unite the nurses in effecting change on their nursing care unit. By cooperating, the nursing staff can bring about changes in their schedules, in patient care assignments and in their roles in assuming responsibility for the nursing care standards of the unit. They do not value Mrs Montoya's leadership skills and will not support her application for the head nurse position.

Miss Sanchez values her employment, good nursing leadership and quality patient care. As a relatively new graduate from nursing school, she does not value the cooperative working relationships of nursing staff as much as her co-workers value them. However, she is aware of the moral obligation for nurses to cooperate with one another for important patient goals. Since the goals of the other nurses are not clear, she is not sure that she is morally obligated to participate with them in airing their views against Mrs Montoya. She realises that her own personal views and goals may become secondary to achieving a greater good for patients, but she is clearly not sure that the planned action of the staff nurse group will actually accomplish good for the patients. In fact, there is a good chance that speaking out against Mrs Montoya will create greater difficulty between the head nurse and staff nurses. The Director of Nursing may also have a negative reaction to the staff nurses' proposed plans.

What is the significance of the conflicts to the parties involved?

Resolving these conflicts of values may be very difficult. Unresolved conflict among staff nurses and their leaders provokes resentment, anger and uncooperative relationships (Corley et al. 2005; Riley & Fry 2000). When these emotions, sentiments and/or attitudes prevail in groups of nurses who must work together, nursing care often becomes haphazard, sometimes barely meeting minimum standards of quality. The focus of the staff becomes the relationships among the staff rather than the patients and the quality of care. Hence, it is always important to resolve conflicting values in planning and initiating nursing care services, otherwise the quality of patient care suffers (Fry & Veatch 2006; Kelly 2006).

The manner in which the conflicting values are resolved may also affect the nurses' job satisfaction, their future career advancement and even their employment status (Wilmot 2000). If the Director of Nursing, Mrs Montoya or anyone else suspects that some nurses are 'troublemakers', they may dismiss the suspected parties or otherwise limit their advancement and/or promotions.

If the nurses are not clear about their goals related to patient care and their reasons for cooperative effort concerning Mrs Montoya's leadership deficits, they may fail to convince the Director of Nursing of their concerns. They may also fail to convince each other of the worthiness of their actions (Hardingham 2004).

What should be done?

The spirit of cooperation among the staff nurses is a positive element that should be strengthened and preserved (Grindel 2006). Cooperating toward mutual goals is supported by the ethical principles of fidelity and beneficence. The nurses should be counselled to continue discussing their views and issues about Mrs Montoya's leadership in staff meetings or in group meetings arranged by the Director of Nursing. There are appropriate means to voice these concerns and they should be discussed directly with Mrs Montoya first. The nurses should also agree on the goals they are promoting and find the best means to express them (Apker et al. 2006).

It is not unusual for a new head nurse to have difficulty gaining the support of the staff. Mrs Montoya needs help in developing the leadership and managerial skills necessary for her new position. The Director of Nursing is responsible for seeing that this help is provided. Seniority on a nursing care unit and expert nursing care knowledge do not always coincide with leadership and managerial skills. Directors of nursing have a responsibility to recognise when staff and newly appointed nurse managers need help in achieving staff nurses' cooperation on matters that affect the quality of patient care and standards of nursing practice (Redman & Fry 2003; Vivar 2006).

The resident physician on this nursing unit can also play an important role by supporting the nurses' motives to create better working conditions and thereby enhance the quality of patient care (Hall et al. 2007). Perhaps there are actions that the resident physician can take to help Mrs Montoya learn the skills important to the head nurse role. By becoming involved in the unit's issues and concerns, physicians can show support for nursing and offer important help in creating co-operation among all staff concerned with patient care.

Since nurses are mandated by society to promote societal good through nursing care activities, the setting in which nursing care takes place is important (Begat, Ellefsen & Severinsson 2005). Certainly every nurse has the opportunity to promote individual good by giving high quality nursing care to the individual patient assigned to her. But if working conditions hamper the ability of the nurse to give expert care or the supply of qualified and competent nurses is inadequate to meet the needs of a group of patients, then individual good may not be a possibility and societal good will eventually suffer.

Working conditions, including inadequate staffing levels, often motivate nurses to join in collective activity or to strike (Aiken, Clarke, Sloane & International Hospital Outcomes Research Consortium 2002). Nurses have engaged in strikes for better working conditions, higher salaries and higher standards of patient care in order to ensure that nurses can meet societal needs for high quality healthcare (Brown et al. 2006; Kovac 2001). Inevitably, nurses often experience serious ethical and legal problems when they engage in strike activities (Loewy 2000; Tabak & Wagner 1997). The following situation demonstrates some of these problems.

Case example 32: When the decision is to strike[2]

What is the story behind the value conflicts?

Clair B, an evening charge nurse, decided to join her fellow nurse co-workers in a strike at their hospital. The decision to strike had been reached several days ago by the majority of nurses in this rehabilitation hospital run by a large corporation. The nurses were seeking higher salaries, fringe benefits and improved working conditions for all nurses employed by the hospital. Clair B had personally experienced many frustrating evenings in the past year due to the loss of nursing staff who became dissatisfied by the long hours and poor salaries. The hospital had tried to fill these vacancies by recruiting nurses from another country and by temporary nurse services. None of the regular nurses were satisfied with the quality of patient care achieved using these approaches.

Now that the strike was imminent, Clair B wondered whether further reducing nursing services for the duration of the strike was in the patients' immediate best interests. Any patient that might suffer from the strike or might be harmed due to care from unfamiliar nursing personnel had already been moved to a special unit where competent nurses would be available who were not participating in the strike. Nonetheless, at least some of the patients on her unit would not do as well with temporary nurses during the strike as they would if their primary nurses remained on the nursing units. The patients would not likely be harmed but they would not necessarily benefit, either. Yet all of the nurses who voted to strike believed they were doing a great service to other nurses in the country and to future patients. By striking, they were helping to make nursing practice more important, more challenging and more desirable. If staff were happier in their jobs and responsible for setting nursing care standards, they reasoned, then future patients would benefit from improved care. Does Clair B have a duty to participate in this kind of action for these reasons?

What is the significance of the values involved?

Providing basic nursing care for the individual patient is an important nursing value, supported by professional mandates and by codes of nursing ethics. Nurses also value the context within which nursing care takes place. If employment conditions, agency regulations or institutional policies create undesirable working conditions that limit the quality of nursing care that can be provided, nurses become concerned (Aiken, Clarke, Sloane, Sochalski & Silber 2002). The quality of nursing care depends, in part, on the environment within which that care takes place. Since nurses value quality of patient care, they also value working conditions that allow and foster quality patient care (Forster et al. 2006).

Clair B is balancing these values as she considers participating in the strike. She values being able to guarantee high quality patient care but realises that in the short term some individual patients may not receive the highest quality nursing care while the strike is in effect. Is this a risk (or loss of benefit) that all patients should be expected to take in return for better patient care in the future? Is safe, but not the highest quality, patient care something that all nurses should be willing to support for the short term in order to obtain a higher standard of patient care for the long term? These are the values in conflict in this case that must be considered by Clair B and the other nurses.

What is the significance of the conflicts to the parties involved?

The profession of nursing places some requirements on its licensed members that can never be set aside (do not kill patients, for example). The obligation to serve the patient, however, can be met in many different ways. One way to serve the individual patient is by collective action to promote a higher quality of nursing care for all patients. The ICN (2004) defines a strike as 'employees' cessation of work or a refusal to work or to continue to work for the purpose of compelling an employer to agree to conditions of work that could not be achieved through negotiation' (p. 1). By making it possible to provide better nursing care to all patients, individual patients will be likely to benefit (Aiken, Clarke, Silber & Sloane 2003). Society will also benefit because a higher standard of nursing care can be expected from all members of the nursing profession. A higher standard eventually becomes a legal as well as a moral requirement of nursing practice.

Some might argue that striking for higher salaries, better fringe benefits and better working conditions achieves benefits for nurses and not patients (Ketter 1997; Loewy 2000). Nurses must keep in mind the principles to be upheld in a strike (Figure 13.1). Certainly, there is no guarantee that improvement in the working conditions of the nurses will result in better patient care and will benefit society. But Clair B and her colleagues argue that poor working conditions reduce nurses' satisfaction with patient care. The best nurses will begin to look for other employment situations while temporary nurses who do not have any loyalty to the institution or to a nursing unit's standard of patient care are hired as replacements. The patients eventually suffer the most because of poor working conditions and the institution's failure to give support to nursing staff for setting nursing care

Position statement – Strike policy

Effective industrial action is compatible with being a health professional so long as essential services are provided. The complete abandonment of ill patients is inconsistent with the purpose and philosophy of professional nurses and their professional organisations as reflected in ICN's *Code of Ethics for Nurses*.

During a strike a minimum essential service to the general public must be maintained.

Other principles to be upheld include:

- Delivery of essential nursing services to a reduced patient population.
- Crisis intervention by nurses for the preservation of life.
- Ongoing nursing care to assure the survival of those unable to care for themselves.
- Nursing care required for therapeutic services without which life would be jeopardised.
- Nursing involvement necessary for urgent diagnostic procedures required to obtain compliance with national/regional legislation as to procedure for implementation of strike action.

Figure 13.1 Excerpts from the ICN Position Statement (ICN 2004).

standards. If nurses cannot control their practice and find institutional supports for quality patient care, they will look for employment elsewhere or provide minimal levels of safe nursing care. Patients may not be overtly harmed by the level of care under such conditions but it is not likely that they will benefit. It is not likely that societal good will be enhanced with this level of nursing care either.

What should be done?

Participating in collective bargaining and well-organised strikes or protests against employers is becoming a legitimate option for nurses. In many countries in the world, nurses gain little recognition for the crucial role they play in the delivery of healthcare. This may be due, in part, to the fact that the majority of nurses are women, a common target of discriminatory employment practices throughout the world. Nonetheless, nurses should be accorded social and economic recognition because they contribute to the general well-being of the citizens by providing essential healthcare services.

By working through their professional organisations, nurses can encourage and promote mechanisms for negotiation between employers, nurses and their representatives. The ICN Position Statement *Socio-economic Welfare of Nurses* (2004) urges all national nursing associations to develop mechanisms to support the negotiating rights of nurses, so that nurses can begin to resolve their employment concerns and engage in collective bargaining as appropriate.

Clair B can assist in promoting standards of nursing care at her hospital by collaborating with her colleagues in striking for better pay and better working conditions. There is no good reason why nurses should receive lower pay, fewer educational opportunities and less chance for promotion than other healthcare workers, just because most nurses are women. If nurses can gain responsibility for, and control over, the quality of nursing care delivered, they will have gained considerable benefit for the health of individual patients and of society in general. This is a morally good goal that can be supported and achieved through nurses' collective actions.

Reporting incompetent nursing care

Nurses have a responsibility to safeguard patients from incompetent and unethical care by any member of the healthcare team. The incompetent healthcare worker may suffer from impairment (i.e. physical or mental illness, substance abuse) or from culpable ignorance of accepted standards of care. The unethical healthcare worker 'knowingly and willingly violates fundamental norms of conduct toward others, especially his or her own patients' (Morreim 1993, p. 19). Nurses should report instances of incompetent and unethical care when they observe or suspect it and know how to follow up a report for the protection of other patients.

Nurses also have a responsibility to participate in patient safety systems and processes, with a view toward reducing the incidence and impact of preventable adverse events (Johnstone 2007a, 2007b; Johnstone & Kanitsaki 2006a). This includes the formal reporting of incidents, including 'honest mistakes' such as medication errors and other errors that can be – and are – often made by even the most conscientious members of staff (Johnstone & Kanitsaki 2005, 2006b).

Unfortunately, documenting human error (honest mistakes), or incompetent and unethical care of another can be difficult. If the nurse has not directly observed an error or an alleged incompetent action, the situation may become that of one person's word against another's. It may also be difficult to determine whether the behaviour or act in question is truly incompetent or an unfortunate mistake that anyone could make.

Morreim (1993) recommends identifying five levels of adverse outcome to patients as a way to distinguish insignificant mishaps from real mistakes that indicate incompetence. The first level of adverse outcome is an accident, which occurs independent of any person's decision or action. It is something that just happens, such as an equipment failure. The second level concerns a well-justified decision that simply turns out badly, such as administering an ordered blood transfusion to which a patient suffers a severe reaction. The adverse outcome does not necessarily indicate that the healthcare worker is incompetent.

At the third level are situations where professionals disagree (there is no consensus on what is the 'right' thing to do) and someone's decision later results in harm to the patient. For example, a nurse might decide to wait and observe the patient longer before reporting troubling symptoms and reactions to the physician. If there are no firm guidelines on what should be reported, when and for what reasons it should be reported, then the matter is left to the nurse's experience and judgment.

The fourth level of adverse outcome is when the healthcare worker exercises poor, although not 'bad', judgment or skill. For example, the nurse may forget to ask the patient if he is currently taking any cardiac medications or fail to observe signs of physical abuse in a paediatric patient. Incompetence should be suspected if the healthcare worker has shown a pattern of such mistakes.

The fifth level of adverse outcome is where true violations of the expected quality of care occur. For example, a nurse may leave a confused, elderly patient unattended in the bathroom. Were the patient to fall and sustain serious injuries, the cause of the incident could be construed as involving a negligent violation of acceptable standards of care.

Evaluating unethical misconduct on the part of a colleague involves a different process to evaluating 'honest errors' and raises slightly different concerns. According to Morreim (1993), the professional must first consider the degree to which the conduct in question violates the accepted standards of the professional group and the expectations of the community. Accepting a small gift from a patient may be acceptable nursing practice in many parts of the world. However, revealing confidential information about a particular patient in a public setting and thereby embarrassing or compromising the patient is not acceptable nursing practice anywhere.

The professional next considers the seriousness of the violation. Is the action always morally wrong for the health professional (for example, engaging in sexual relations with a patient)? Has the action harmed the patient (for example, informing an employer of an employee's positive HIV status, resulting in loss of the employee's job)?

These guidelines offer the nurse a starting point for evaluating questionable actions or behaviours by co-workers to determine whether they are either incompetent or unethical. They help the nurse to decide whether it is appropriate to take action against a co-worker. Even when a colleague's behaviour is clearly incompetent or unethical, it is very difficult to report someone with whom you work closely or whose personal problems might contribute to incompetent or unethical conduct. The following case example shows how one nurse was confronted with the need to report a nursing colleague.

Exercise:

Case example 33: Reporting a colleague to protect the patient[3]

What is the story behind the value conflicts?

Rebecca Fein and Sarah Goldman were staff nurses on the night shift in a paediatric surgical unit. One night, as they neared the completion of their shift, Miss Fein noted that a 6-year-old diabetic patient recovering from minor surgery looked very pale and was perspiring. When she was unable to awaken the patient, she notified her colleague and best friend Miss Goldman, and together they did a blood sugar test. The results confirmed Miss Fein's fears: the child was in hypoglycaemic coma. They called the physician and the patient was immediately transferred to the intensive care unit. The child recovered and was discharged home within a week.

Later, Miss Fein reviewed the incident, stating how surprised she was to find the child in a hypoglycaemic state. At first Miss Goldman did not say much but finally admitted that it was all her fault. She had miscalculated the child's insulin dose and had given her too much medication. She had not gone back to check on the child and only realised her mistake when Miss Fein found the child in a hypoglycaemic state.

Miss Fein was shocked and asked whether her friend had completed an incident report or notified the child's physician. Miss Goldman said she did not intend to report it because that would create an inquiry and trouble for her. 'I can do without that right now', she stated. She was being considered for an advancement in the clinical ladder programme of the nursing division and feared that the incident would reflect unfavourably on her employment record. She looked at Miss Fein and said meaningfully, '. . . and I hope you're not going to report it, either. I told you this in confidence and as a friend, and it would be unethical for you to do anything about it.' What should Miss Fein do?

Discussion questions

What is the significance of the values involved?

(1) What values are being expressed by Miss Goldman? Which values seem to hold more meaning or importance for her?
(2) What values are all nurses presumed to hold concerning honest errors/ mistakes in providing nursing care?
(3) What values are patients presumed to hold about their care?
(4) What values does the organisation hold in regard to clinical risk management and patient safety systems and processes?
(5) Which ethical principles seem to apply to this case example? What does it mean to avoid harming the patient?
(6) How does the moral concept of accountability apply to this case? What does it mean for Miss Fein to be accountable? For Miss Goldman to be accountable?

What is the significance of the conflicts to the parties involved?

(7) Are the conflicts of values in this case significant? For nursing practice? For patient health and welfare? For the nurses' employment records?
(8) How might the value conflicts affect nursing practice? Future patient care?
(9) What are the relevant standards for nursing practice in this case?
(10) What ethical requirements of nursing practice provide guidance in this case?
(11) What is the level of 'adverse outcome' that occurs in this case?

What should be done?

(12) What are Miss Goldman's moral responsibilities in the case?
(13) What are Miss Fein's moral responsibilities in the case? Is she dealing with an honest error or incompetent or unethical practice, or a combination of all three?
(14) To what extent should personal friendship affect a nurse's judgment about reporting an honest mistake, incompetent and/or unethical practice?

(15) What course of action would you take if you were Miss Fein?

(16) How would you support your judgment or action by ethical principles and concepts of nursing?

Summary

The moral obligation to protect the patient from harm is a strong one in nursing practice. When the judgments or actions of others endanger the patient or the patient's health, the nurse must report these judgments or actions to superiors. In some cases, the nurse may need to act at once to protect the patient from harms that may occur before others can intervene. This responsibility may be hard to carry out when the offending actions are made by physicians or by co-workers who are also friends. For a variety of reasons, nurses may feel pressured not to report actions that endanger the patient. They may also experience stress and conflict with other nursing personnel as a result of reporting actions. However, the ethical obligation to protect the patient from preventable adverse events, incompetent and/or unethical actions that endanger the individual patient or the quality of care to many patients is very clear.

Likewise, when the delivery of patient care is affected by organisational disorganisation or working conditions that prevent optimal nursing practice, the nurse may need to collaborate with co-workers to bring about change. While nurses sometimes strike for improved working conditions as well as personal benefits, the goal is to enhance nurses' abilities to provide patient care.

Notes

1 Adapted from Tate, B.L. (1977) *The nurse's dilemma: Ethical considerations in nursing practice*. Geneva, Switzerland: ICN (p. 57). Used with permission.
2 Adapted from Fry, S.T. & Veatch, R.M. (2006) *Case studies in nursing ethics*, 3rd ed. Boston, Jones & Bartlett Publishers (pp. 88–89). Used with permission.
3 Adapted from Carlisle, D. (1991) Protecting patients. *Nursing Times* 97(8), 52.

References

Aiken, L.H., Clarke, S.P., Sloane, D.M. & International Hospital Outcomes Research Consortium (2002) *Int J Qual Health Care* 14(1), 5–13.
Aiken, L.H., Clarke, S.P., Sloane, D.M., Sochalski, J. & Silber, J.H. (2002) Hospital nurse staffing and patient mortality, nurse burnout, and job dissatisfaction. *JAMA* 288(16), 1987–1992.
Aiken, L.H., Clarke, S.P., Silber, J.H. & Sloane, D. (2003) Hospital nurse staffing, education, and patient mortality. *LDI Issue Brief* 9(2), 1–4.
Apker, J., Propp, K.M., Zabava Ford, W.S. & Hofmeister, N. (2006) Collaboration, credibility, compassion, and coordination: Professional nurse communication skillsets in health care team interactions. *J Prof Nurs* 22(3), 180–189.

Arndt, M. (1999) The ethical issues with which nurses grapple are often brought to a point by polarizing the interests of nurses against those of doctors. *Nurs Ethics* 6(6), 449–450.

Ashworth, P. (2000) Nurse–doctor relationships: Conflict, competition or collaboration. *Intensive Crit Care Nurs* 16, 127–128.

Begat, I., Ellefsen, B. & Severinsson, E. (2005) Nurses' satisfaction with their work environment and the outcomes of clinical nursing supervision on nurses' experiences of well-being – a Norwegian study. *J Nurs Manag* 13(3), 221–230.

Brown, G.D., Greaney, A.M., Kelly-Fitzgibbon, M.E. & McCarthy, J. (2006) The 1999 Irish nurses' strike: Nursing versions of the strike and self-identity in a general hospital. *J Adv Nurs* 56(2), 200–208.

Castledine, G. (2004) Nurses must learn methods to deal with difficult doctors. *Br J Nurs* 13(8), 479.

Corley, J.C., Minick, P., Elswick, R.K. & Jacobs, M. (2005) Nurse moral distress and ethical work environment. *Nurs Ethics* 12(4), 381–390.

Davidhizar, R. & Dowd, S. (2003) The doctor–nurse relationship. *J Pract Nurs* 53(4), 9–12.

Forster, D.A., McLachlan, J.L., Yelland, J., Rayner, J., Lumley, J. & Davey, M.A. (2006) Staffing in postnatal units: Is it adequate for the provision of quality care: Staff perspectives from a state-wide review of postnatal care in Victoria, Australia. *BMC Health Serv Res* 6(83) (4 July).

Fry, S.T. (2004) Nursing ethics. In S.G. Post (Ed) *Encyclopedia of bioethics*, 3rd ed. (1898–1903). New York: Macmillan Reference USA: Thomson/Gale.

Fry, S.T. & Veatch, R.M. (2006) *Case studies in nursing ethics*, 3rd ed. Boston: Jones and Bartlett.

Grindel, C. (2006) The nurse's responsibility in creating a 'nurse-friendly' culture in the workplace. *Medsurg Nurs* 15(3), 125–126.

Hall, P., Weaver, L., Gravelle, D. & Thibault, H. (2007) Developing collaborative person-centered practice: A pilot project on a palliative care unit. *J Interprof Care* 21(1), 69–81.

Hardingham, L.B. (2004) Integrity and moral residue: Nurses as participants in a moral community. *Nurs Philos* 5(2), 127–134.

Homsted, L. (2003) Nurse/physician communication. *Fla Nurse* 51(1), 4.

Iacono, M. (2003) Conflict, communication, and collaboration: Improving interactions between nurses and physicians. *J Perianesth Nurs* 18(1), 42–46.

International Council of Nurses (ICN) (1999) *Position statement: Strike policy.* Geneva: ICN.

International Council of Nurses (ICN) (2000) *Position statement: Rights of children.* Geneva, ICN.

International Council of Nurses (ICN) (2004) *Position statement: Socio-economic welfare of nurses.* Geneva, ICN.

International Council of Nurses (ICN) (2006) *Code of ethics for nurses.* Geneva ICN.

Johnstone, M. (2007a) Patient safety ethics and human error management in ED contexts, Part I: Development of the global patient safety movement. *Australasian Emergency Nurses Journal* 10(1), 13–20.

Johnstone, M. (2007b) Patient safety ethics and human error management in ED contexts, Part II: Accountability and the challenge to change. *Australasian Emergency Nurses Journal* 10(2), 80–85.

Johnstone, M. & Kanitsaki, O. (2005) Processes for disciplining nurses for unprofessional conduct of a 'serious' nature: a critique. *Journal of Advanced Nursing* 50(4), 363–371.

Johnstone, M. & Kanitsaki, O. (2006a) The moral imperative of designating patient safety and quality care a national nursing research priority. *Collegian* 13(1), 5–9.

Johnstone, M. & Kanitsaki, O. (2006b) The ethics and practical importance of defining, distinguishing and disclosing nursing errors: a discussion paper. *International Journal of Nursing Studies* 43(3), 367–376.

Kelly, J. (2006) An overview of conflict. *Dimens Crit Care Nurs* 25(1), 22–28.

Ketter, J. (1997) Nurses and strikes: A perspective from the United States. *Nurs Ethics* 4(4), 323–329.

Kovac, C. (2001) Polish nurses strike for better wages. *BMJ* 322(7277), 10.

LeTourneau, B. (2004) Physicians and nurses: Friends or foes? *J Healthc Manag* 49(1), 12–15.

Loewy, R.H. (2000) Of healthcare professionals, ethics, and strikes. *Camb Q Healthc Ethics* 9(4), 513–520.

Marrone, C. (2003) Home health care nurses' perceptions of physician–nurse relationships. *Qual Health Res* 13(5), 623–635.

Morreim, E.H. (1993) Am I my brother's warden? Responding to the unethical or incompetent colleague. *Hast Ctr Rep* 23(3), 19–27.

Oberle, K. & Hughes, D. (2001) Doctors' and nurses' perceptions of ethical problems in end-of-life decisions. *J Adv Nurs* 33(6), 707–715.

Redman, B.A. & Fry, S.T. (2003) Ethics and human rights issues experienced by nurses in leadership roles. *Nurs Leadersh Forum* 7(4), 150–156.

Riley, J.M. & Fry, S.T. (2000) Troubled advocacy: nurses report widespread ethical conflicts. *Reflections on Nursing Leadership*, 2nd Qtr, 35–36, 45.

Stein, L.I. (1967) The doctor–nurse game. *Arch Gen Psych* 16, 699–703.

Stein, L.I., Watts, D.T. & Howell, T. (1990) The doctor–nurse game revisited. *Nurs Outlook* 38(6), 264–268.

Tabak, N. & Orit, K. (2007) Relationship between how nurses resolve their conflicts with doctors, their stress and job satisfaction. *J Nurs Man* 15(3), 321–331.

Tabak, N. & Wagner, N. (1997) Professional solidarity versus responsibility for the health of the public: Is a nurses' strike morally defensible? *Nurs Ethics* 4(4), 283–293.

Vivar, C.G. (2006) Putting conflict management into practice: A nursing case study. *J Nurs Manag* 14(3), 201–206.

Wilmot, S. (2000) Nurses and whistleblowing: The ethical issues. *J Adv Nurs* 32(5), 1051–1057.

Appendix 1
Teaching ethics to nurses

Sara T. Fry

Formerly, Henry R. Luce Professor of Nursing Ethics
Boston College School of Nursing
Chestnut Hill, MA, USA

Many forms of ethics teaching within schools of nursing have evolved over the years. Early textbooks written by physicians, religious advisors and nurse leaders usually included content on ethics and etiquette as both were considered essential to ethical nurse behaviours (Aikens 1931; Gladwin 1930; Robb 1921). In the 1970s, however, changes in the delivery of healthcare, the use of new technologies, the expanding role of the nurse, and changing social conditions raised the question: Are nurses adequately prepared for complex ethical decision making in their new and more responsible roles in healthcare?

To answer this question, researchers began to analyse how ethics was taught in schools of nursing. A study of ethics teaching in 209 accredited baccalaureate nursing programmes in the United States of America revealed that general ethics content was integrated in the curricula of two-thirds of the programmes surveyed (Aroskar 1977). Twenty years later, this finding was confirmed in a study of over 2000 registered nurses practising in six New England states (Fry & Duffy 2001), and in a study of 398 registered and enrolled nurses in Victoria, Australia (Johnstone, DaCosta & Turale 2004). In the study of New England nurses, 58% of the RNs surveyed reported having ethics content integrated throughout their nursing educational programmes. In the study of Australian nurses, 80% of the nurses surveyed reported having ethics content integrated throughout their nursing education. In all three studies (Aroskar 1977; Fry & Duffy 2001;

Johnstone, DaCosta & Turale 2004) a high perceived need for the teaching of specific nursing ethics content was reported. Indeed, a study of ethics teaching in programmes of nursing, midwifery and health visiting throughout the UK showed that more than 90% of the programmes surveyed felt that the study of ethics should be part of any nursing curriculum (Gallagher & Boyd 1991). Now, all nursing curricula in the UK are reported to include ethics content (Nolan & Markert 2002).

Given the perceived need for ethics education expressed by both practising nurses and nurse educators over the years, the purpose and content of such ethics education has been at issue (Begley 2006; Dinc & Gorgulu 2002; Doane, Pauly, Brown & McPherson 2004; Gastmans 2002; Woods 2005).

Purpose of teaching ethics to nurses

Early textbooks on nursing ethics clearly describe that the purpose of teaching ethics is to enhance nurses' abilities to:

(1) analyse ethical conflicts encountered in practice, and
(2) make more informed ethical decisions

To achieve this purpose, models for ethical analysis and nurses' ethical decision making were proposed (Bandman & Bandman 1978; Benjamin & Curtis 1992; Bergman 1973; Curtin 1978). These early textbooks often used a case study approach to demonstrate the analysis of ethical conflicts faced by the nurse and to apply ethical decision making models or frameworks to actual patient care situations. The cases studies in these texts tend to support the notion that the most common ethical problems experienced by nurses involve the balancing of harms and benefits in patient care, the protection of patients' dignity and well-being, the distribution of nursing care resources, and cooperative relationships with co-workers, especially the physician (Fry & Veatch 2006).

Over time, there has been a clear consensus that the overall goal of teaching ethics to nurses is to produce a morally accountable practitioner who is skilled in ethical decision making (Fry 2004). Intermediate goals of ethics teaching are to:

● examine personal commitments and values in relation to the care of patients
● engage in ethical reflection
● develop skill in moral reasoning and moral judgment
● develop the ability to use ethics for reflection on broader issues having policy implications and for research on the moral foundations of practice

In the 1980s, however, the need for a coherent approach to the integrated teaching of ethics in nursing curricula has been recognised (Ryden, Duckett, Crisham, Caplan & Schmitz 1989) along with the need to set different goals for the teaching of ethics in undergraduate, master's and doctoral nursing programmes (Ketefian 1999).

Approaches to teaching ethics

Contemporary approaches to teaching ethics include the integration of ethics content throughout the programme of nursing, and ethics content in an identified course on nursing ethics or healthcare ethics. The latter method usually focuses on the ethical concepts of nursing practice or the ethical issues that arise in nursing practice. Other approaches to teaching ethics include the development of intuition and moral imagination. Each of these approaches will be described below.

Integrated ethics content approach

An integrated curriculum attempts to weave an identifiable strand of content throughout a programme of study (Duckett, Waithe, Rowan, Schmitz & Ryden 1993). Where ethics content is concerned, the domain of ethics is clearly identified and then carefully sequenced from course to course in the various levels of the programme in order to enhance student development and to build on previous learning experiences. The advantages of an integrated approach to ethics teaching include avoidance of undesirable duplication of content and avoidance of gaps in learning. The ethics content is also introduced to the student when it is most applicable throughout student progression in the programme.

One of the best examples of an integrated ethics curriculum has been developed at the University of Minnesota School of Nursing (Duckett & Ryden 1994; Duckett, Waithe, Rowan, Schmitz & Ryden 1993; Ryden et al. 1989). As described by Ryden and her colleagues (1989, p. 105), the overall objectives for this ethics programme of study are to:

- appreciate the nature and complexity of ethical issues in the practice of nursing
- articulate an evolving personal ethical philosophy and relate it to an evolving philosophy of nursing
- describe resources, relevant to ethics, such as committees, organisations and media, indicating how these might be used in professional development and practice
- make ethical decisions after critically analysing the situation and applying ethical principles, theories and codes
- take actions which are congruent with the ethical decision
- evaluate the relationship between the student's own personal ethical philosophy and his or her personal and professional behaviour
- progress in level of moral reasoning toward more principled reasoning
- recognise the independent responsibility of the nurse with respect to ethical concerns in practice

The educational strategies used in the programme are based on the four components of moral behaviour (i.e., moral sensitivity, moral reasoning, moral commitment and moral action) identified by Rest (1982). Reports of the programme indicate

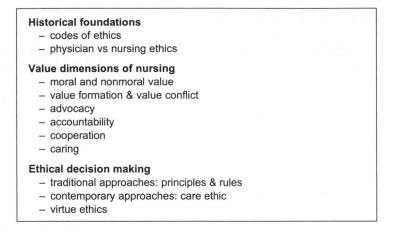

Figure A1-1   Ethical concepts approach to ethics teaching.

that students progressively increased their moral reasoning abilities throughout the programme of ethics education (Duckett, Rowan, Ryden, Krichbaum, Miller, Wainwright & Savik 1997).

Ethical concepts approach

Course content based on this method of ethics teaching usually begins with the historical foundations of the nursing ethic as found in the writings of nursing's early leaders (Figure A1-1). For example, readings from Nightingale (1859), Robb (1921), Aikens (1931) and Gladwin (1930) would be discussed to distinguish ethics from etiquette in nursing practice. Historical documents on the need for a code of ethics in nursing practice would also be discussed. The need for a code of ethics is well documented in nursing journals and other nursing documents from the early 1900s. It would be important to trace the development of the ICN *Code of Ethics for Nurses* (2006) including its various forms to the present time. Comparison of the ICN *Code of Ethics for Nurses* with other codes, particularly codes of ethical practice for physicians and other health workers, should be made. Additionally, other normative statements of the professions (for example, the Hippocratic Oath and the Florence Nightingale Pledge), should be read and reviewed.

By discussing the differences between the development of codes of ethics for the practice of medicine and the practice of nursing, important distinctions between physician and nursing ethics are made evident. Understanding the distinctions usually gives nursing students greater respect for, and understanding of, the values of both medicine and nursing. This respect and understanding are essential to the effective collaboration of nurses, physicians and other health professionals.

The major focus in the ethical concepts approach to ethics teaching is the value dimensions of nursing. The nature of values and value conflicts are explored and the differences between moral and nonmoral values are emphasised. These distinctions are important to make because ethical conflicts contain conflicts over moral values (Romyn 2003). Students need to have formal knowledge about the meaning of values and how values are expressed in healthcare systems of care. They also need to know the value foundations of professional nursing and be able to recognise how these values often conflict with those of healthcare institutions and even society (Glen 1999; Lemonidou, Papathanassoglou, Giannakipoulou, Patiraki & Papadatou 2004). Last, effective interprofessional collaboration often depends on respecting differences in values and beliefs when responding to patient care needs (Fry & Veatch 2006).

The ethical concepts approach also includes content on the types of ethical problems that are commonly experienced in nursing practice. According to Jameton (1984), the first type of ethical problem is one of 'moral uncertainty'. This is the type of situation in which the nurse is unsure about the moral problem at issue and which moral values or ethical principles are involved.

The second type of ethical problem is that of 'moral dilemma.' This is the type of situation that arises when two or more ethical principles seem to apply to the situation but they support mutually inconsistent courses of action for the nurse. Faced with this type of situation, the nurse is truly in a 'dilemma' in terms of choices of action.

The third type of ethical problem is that of 'moral distress.' This situation arises when the nurse knows the moral values at issue, knows the ethical principles that ought to guide action and has chosen the right course of action based on these values and principles. However, the nurse cannot do the right action because she is constrained from doing so. Constraints may include a lack of power or decision-making authority, institutional rules and authority over the nurse, or even lack of respect for the nurse's role in decision making. Moral distress has become a common form of ethical conflict for the nurse in recent years (Cohen & Erickson 2006; Corley, Minick, Elswick & Jacobs 2005; Rushton 2006).

These descriptions of the ethical problems experienced by nurses make it easy to see that the majority of conflicts that nurses describe as an 'ethical dilemma' are very complex problems. They often contain administrative, communicative and even legal dimensions. Yet, the ability to sort out the ethical aspects from the other aspects in a patient care situation is very important to the development of ethical decision-making skill.

Teaching ethics by focusing on the ethical concepts provides students with the opportunity to test their understanding by analysing and discussing carefully, chosen patient care situations involving nursing care. Once the student can decipher the different values at issue in a patient care situation, he or she begins to understand the nature of value conflicts. The values of nurses, patients, family members, physicians and institutions are analysed and the nature of ethical obligation is discussed. The patient care situations give the student experience in moral reasoning and demonstrate the role of values in nurses' ethical decision making.

The ethical concepts method of teaching usually includes a description of traditional forms of ethical reasoning and the application of ethical rules and principles to types of situations (Bebeau 2002). This is important because the application of ethical rules and principles needs to be integrated with other approaches to ethical decision making (Auvinen, Suominen, Leino-Kilpi & Helkama 2004; Kim, Park, Son & Han 2004; Nolan & Markert 2002). Ethics is not merely the application of a 'formula' of accepted rules, principles and theories whenever ethical conflicts arise in patient care. The acceptance and understanding of different value orientations, knowledge of the discipline of ethics and ethical skill all play a role in making decisions about patient care.

It is also helpful to include some content on virtue ethics which goes beyond the application of principles and rules. Virtue ethics considers the motives of the decision maker and the development of moral character (Begley 2006). It is a form of ethics that helps one to know how and when to put ethical rules and principles to work. As a form of normative ethics, virtue ethics offers an account of the kind of persons nurses ought to be and not just what one ought to do in the role of nurse. Combining virtue ethics with the other aspects of ethical decision making seems to make very good sense for the practice of nursing.

Ethical issues approach

This approach to ethics teaching focuses on ethical issues that arise in nursing practice (Figure A1-2). These are the issues that usually dominate the newspaper headlines and have become concerns of all members of society. Termination of life-sustaining treatments, abortion, surrogate motherhood, in vitro fertilisation, euthanasia, assisted suicide, allocation of scarce healthcare resources and the treatment of severely disabled infants and intellectually disabled adults are topics of moral concern that are best discussed in courses designed for this purpose. By discussing these issues, the growth of bioethics as a discipline, and the development of public opinion on matters of ethical concern are made evident. It is also helpful for students to read any published reports and policy recommendations concerning the issues. Discussions of historic legal cases demonstrate both legal

---

Approach to ethical issues
- historical development of the issue
- legal and policy dimensions

Ethical issues
- termination of treatment decisions
- abortion
- in vitro fertilisation
- surrogate motherhood
- euthanasia & assisted suicide
- allocation of scarce resources
- treatment of disabled infants and the mentally retarded

Figure A1-2 Ethical issues approach to ethics teaching.

and ethical dimensions of an issue from country to country. The abortion issue is one in which classic ethical positions were formulated that subsequently influenced the development of legal judgments on abortion and on other issues – termination of treatment decisions, for example.

There are several advantages to the ethical issues approach to teaching. The approach can be easily adapted and changed depending on the issues to be discussed. The various issues can be taught as separate modules in basic nursing education in clinical courses (Kalvemark, Hoglund, Hansson, Westerholm & Arnetz 2004). It can also be easily adapted to continuing education offerings in ethics and is often the preferred approach for short conferences, one-day workshops, and in-service education programmes. It is also the typical teaching approach of academic courses offered by philosophy departments (Webb & Warwick 1999).

Other approaches to teaching ethics

Development of intuition

One additional approach to teaching ethics emphasises the development of intuition as a way of moral knowing (Effken 2001). Intuitive thinking 'has certain essential features and involves the use of a sound, rational, relevant knowledge base in situations that, through experience, are so familiar that the person has learned how to recognise and act on appropriate patterns' (Easen & Wilcockson 1996, p. 667).

One feature of intuition is a nonconscious recognition of, awareness of or insight into a situation. A second feature of intuition is that it stems from a deep involvement in an issue or problem. A third feature of intuition is that it is spontaneous and often defies explanation. These features are usually present in intuitions resulting from a knowledge base (often called tacit knowledge) and from experience (White 2006). The person with the intuition thus perceives a situation by recognising patterns within the situation (McCutcheon & Pincombe 2001). The intuiter makes sense of the situation in a way that leads to a decision, using nonlinear methods of reasoning considered valid in that they are based on knowledge and experience.

Just as intuitive knowing is recognised as a component of professional nursing expertise (Effken 2001; Tanner, Benner, Chesla & Gordon 1996), it is also being recognised as an important part of moral excellence in nursing practice. Including within ethics education educational strategies that enhance the development of intuition is thus encouraged.

Development of imagination

A second nontraditional approach to teaching ethics involves the development of the imagination (Maxwell 2005). It is based on the belief that the imaginative capacity of the nurse plays an important part in:

(1)   the quality of the nurse's role enactment
(2)   the moral strategies that the nurse uses in practice
(3)   the nurse's ability to communicate in patient care
(4)   the type of person that the nurse becomes (Scott 1997)

The moral imagination is believed to facilitate moral knowing and the understanding of a situation. It is even considered by some to be necessary for the ability to have empathy toward a patient or to be able 'to understand and imaginatively enter into another person's feelings' or world (Scott 1997, p. 46).

To be effective, strategies that stimulate the moral imagination require that the student first be a person of good character. Once good character is assured, the moral imagination can be effectively stimulated through the use of the humanities, especially the reading of literature (Begley 2006). Such reading will develop moral sensitivity and moral imagination by inviting the reader to go beyond his or her immediate experience to that of others and to consider the common bonds of humanity between the reader and the characters in the work of literature. Reading poetry and short stories, as well as viewing videos and art, can have the same effect on the student. Nursing ethics education that includes experiences to enhance the moral imagination is thus encouraged.

Clinical ethics teaching strategies

Over the years, good clinical ethics teaching strategies have been developed. These strategies are similar to traditional clinical teaching strategies for nursing practice, and use the clinical setting rather than the classroom. They promise to influence positively how students interact with their patients in discussing their ethical concerns (Kalvemark, Hoglund, Hansson, Westerholm & Arnetz 2004). Teaching is characterised by informal instruction rather than formal course outlines, lectures and written evaluation methods. These strategies are the clinical conference, the case study presentation and ethics rounds (Figure A1-3).

The clinical conference

This ethics teaching strategy involves a presentation on an ethical issue that affects patient care (i.e., termination of treatment, selective termination of pregnancy, organ retrieval from anencephalic newborns), followed by discussion in an interdisciplinary context. The issue selected for discussion is usually related to

Clinical conference
Case study presentation
Ethics rounds

Figure A1-3   Clinical ethics teaching strategies.

the clinical area holding the conference (critical care, obstetrics, neonatal intensive care, etc.). The relevant ethical, legal and social dimensions of the issue are discussed and various arguments for and against the issue are presented. Institutional policy about the issue may be discussed or policy recommendations are made that can be implemented at a later date. Ethics learning occurs through the examination of ethical positions on the issue and the application of ethical thought in policy recommendations.

The case study presentation

This ethics teaching strategy is carried out with a small group of students or practitioners. The instructor must understand the extent of previous clinical and academic experiences of the group members and their knowledge of ethics. The patient care situation is carefully chosen by the instructor to demonstrate the human dimensions of an ethical conflict by focusing on the values of patients, nurses and other healthcare workers. This teaching strategy helps the student to analyse the nature of the ethical problem in this situation and distinguish the moral values from the nonmoral values involved. This strategy emphasises the roles that nurses play in ethical decision making. It is an excellent approach to use with students in their initial exposure to the clinical setting because it sensitises students to how nurses function in clinical situations. It also illustrates the types of ethical decisions that nurses commonly make.

Ethics rounds

The use of ethics rounds with nurses in clinical settings is a relatively new strategy for teaching ethics. It uses traditional clinical rounds teaching with a focus on the ethical dimensions of patient care rather than on clinical diagnosis and treatment.

As with the case study presentation, ethics rounds requires careful selection of patients to be presented and discussed. Unlike the case study presentation, in ethics rounds the instructor speaks directly to the patient, and to family members, and may even hold the discussion at the bedside. To do this, of course, the instructor must obtain consent from the patient.

Ethics rounds is an excellent ethics teaching strategy because it is interdisciplinary. House staff, staff nurses and students are all usually involved. Anyone who is skilled in ethical decision making can do the presentation of the patients and the ethical issues. Students are asked questions about the nature and scope of the ethical problem, the types of arguments for and against options, and are urged to come to some consensus, with the patient, on the actions chosen.

One advantage of the ethics rounds approach is that it exposes the student to the culture of the clinical setting. Students learn how those who work together often rely on one another in providing optimal patient care. Open discussion among students and clinicians fosters the cooperative relationships among healthcare workers and aids the transition from student to clinician. This method gives the student experience in openly discussing an ethical question related to patient care and in presenting his or her own view on the matter. It incorporates elements of ethics consultation into ethics rounds and thus results in a more comprehensive approach to ethics learning (Boisaubin and Carter 1999). By actually going through the process of an ethical analysis with the patient, the student gains communication skills that will increase his or her decision-making ability. As Benner (1984) points out, such experiences often serve as important exemplars for future situations that the nurse might confront.

References

Aikens, C. (1931) *Studies in ethics for nurses.* Philadelphia: W.B. Saunders.

Aroskar, M.A. (1977) Ethics in the nursing curriculum. *Nursing Outlook*, 25(4), 260–264.

Auvinen, J., Suominen, T., Leino-Kilpi, H. & Helkama, K. (2004) The development of moral judgment during nursing education in Finland. *Nurse Educ Today* 24(7), 538–546.

Bandman, B. & Bandman, E. (Eds) (1978) *Bioethics and human rights: A reader for health professionals.* Boston: Little-Brown.

Bebeau, M.J. (2002) The defining issues test and the four component model: Contributions to professional education. *J Moral Educ* 31(3), 271–295.

Begley, A.M. (2006) Facilitating the development of moral insight in practice: Teaching ethics and teaching virtue. *Nurs Philos* 7(4), 257–265.

Benjamin M. & Curtis, J. (1992) *Ethics in nursing*, 3rd ed. New York: Oxford University Press.

Benner, P. (1984) *From novice to expert: Excellence and power in clinical nursing practice.* Menlo Park, CA: Addison-Wesley.

Bergman, R. (1973) Evolving ethical concepts for nursing. *International Nursing Review*, 23(4), 116–117.

Boisaubin, E.V. & Carter, M.A. (1999) Optimizing ethics services and educaiton in a teaching hospital: Rounds versus consultation. *The Journal of Clinical Ethics*, 10(4), 294–299.

Cohen, J.S. & Erickson, J.J. (2006) Ethical dilemmas and moral distress in oncology nursing practice. *Clin J Oncol Nurs* 10(6), 775–780.

Corley, M.C., Minick, P., Elswick, R.K. & Jacobs, M. (2005) Nurse moral distress and ethical work environment. *Nurs Ethics* 12(4), 381–390.

Curtin, L. (1978) A proposed model for critical ethical analysis. *Nursing Forum*, 17, 12–17.

Davis, A.J., Tschudin, V. & DeRaeve, L. (Eds) (2006) *Essentials of teaching and learning in nursing ethics: Perspectives and methods.* Edinburgh/New York: Churchill Livingstone Elsevier.

Dinc, L. & Gorgulu, R.S. (2002) Teaching ethics in nursing. *Nurs Ethics* 9(3), 259–268.

Doane, G., Pauly, B., Brown, H. & McPherson, G. (2004) Exploring the heart of ethical nursing practice: Implications for ethics education. *Nurs Ethics* 11(3), 240–253.

Duckett, L., Rowan, M., Ryden, M., Krichbaum, K., Miller, M., Wainwright, H. & Savik, K. (1997) Progress in the moral reasoning of baccalaureate nursing students between program entry and exit. *Nursing Research*, 46(4), 222–228.

Duckett, L. & Ryden, M. (1994) Education for ethical nusing practice. In J. Rest & D. Narvaez (Eds) *Moral development in the professions* (pp. 51–69). Hillsdale, NJ: Erlbaum.

Duckett, L., Waithe, M.E., Rowan, M., Schmitz, L. & Ryden, M. (1993) *MCSL building: Developing a strong ethics curriculum in nursing using multi-course sequential learning*, 2nd ed. Minneapolis, MN: University of Minnesota School of Nursing.

Easen, P. & Wilcockson, J. (1996) Intuition and rational decision-making in professional thinking: A false dichotomy? *Journal of Advanced Nursing* 24, 667–673.

Effken, J.A. (2001) Informational basis for expert intuition. *J Adv Nurs* 34(2), 246–255.

Fry, S.T. (1989) Teaching ethics in nursing curricula: Traditional and contemporary models. *Nursing Clinics of North America* 24(2), 485–497.

Fry, S.T. (2004) Nursing ethics. In S.G. Post (Ed) *Encyclopedia of bioethics*, 3rd ed (pp. 1898–1903). New York: Macmillian Reference, USA.

Fry, S.T. & Duffy, M.E. (2001) The development and psychometric evaluation of the Ethical Issues Scale (EIS). *Journal of Nursing Scholarship* 33(3), 273–277.

Fry, S.T. & Veatch, R.M. (2006) *Case studies in nursing ethic*, 3rd ed. Boston: Jones & Bartlett, Publishers.

Gallagher, U. & Boyd, K.M. (1991) *Teaching and learning: Nursing ethics*. Middlesex, England: Scutari Press.

Gastmans, C. (2002) A fundamental ethical approach to nursing: Some proposals for ethics education. *Nurs Ethics* 9(5), 494–507.

Gladwin, M.E. (1930) *Ethics: Talks to nurses*. Philadelphia: W.B. Saunders.

Glen, S. (1999) Educating for interprofessional collaboration: Teaching about values. *Nurs Ethics* 6(3), 202–213.

International Council of Nurses (ICN) (2006) *Code of ethics for nurses*. Geneva, Switzerland: ICN.

Jameton, A. (1984) *Nursing practice: The ethical issues*. Englewood Cliffs, NJ: Prentice-Hall.

Johnstone, M., DaCosta, C. & Turale, S. (2004) Registered and enrolled nurses' experiences of ethical issues in nursing practice. *Australian Journal of Advanced Nursing* 22(1), 31–37.

Kalvemark, S., Hoglund, A.T., Hansson, M.G., Westerholm, P. & Arnetz, B. (2004) Living with conflicts – ethical dilemmas and moral distress in the health care system. *Soc Sci Med* 58(6), 1075–1085.

Ketefian, S. (1999) Ethics content in nursing education. *Journal of Professional Nursing* 15(3), 138.

Kim, Y.S., Park, J.W., Son, Y.J. & Han, S.S. (2004) A longitudinal study on the development of moral judgement in Korean nursing students. *Nurs Ethics* 11(3), 254–265.

Lemonidou, D., Papathanassoglou, E., Giannakopoulou, M., Patiraki, E. & Papadatou, D. (2004) Moral professional personhood: Ethical reflections during initial clinical encounters in nursing education. *Nurs Ethics* 11(2), 122–137.

Maxwell, B. (2005) Imitation, imagination, and re-appraisal: Educating the moral emotions. *J of Moral Educ* 34(3), 291–307.

McCutcheon, H.H.I. & Pincombe, J. (2001) Intuition: An important tool in the practice of nursing. *J Adv Nurs* 35(3), 342–348.

Nightingale, F. (1859) *Notes on nursing: What it is, and what it is not*. London, England: Harrison & Sons.

Nolan, P.W. & Markert, D. (2002) Ethical reasoning observed: A longitudinal study of nursing students. *Nurs Ethics* 9(3), 243–258.

Rest, J. (1982) A psychologist looks at the teaching of ethics. *Hast Ctr Rprt*, 12(1), 29–36.

Robb, I.H. (1921) *Nursing ethics: For hospital and private use*. Cleveland: E.C. Loeckert.

Romyn, D.M. (2003) The relational narrative: Implications for nurse practice and education. *Nurs Philos* 4(2), 149–154.

Rudnick, A. (2002) The ground of dialogical bioethics. *Health Care Anal* 10(4), 391–402.

Rushton, C.H. (2006) Defining and addressing moral distress: Tools for critical care nursing leaders. *AACN Adv Crit Care* 17(2), 161–168.

Ryden, M.B., Duckett, L., Crisham, P., Caplan, A. & Schmitz, K. (1989) Multi-course sequential learning as a model for content integration: Ethics as a prototype. *Journal of Nursing Education* 28(3), 102–106.

Scott, P.A. (1997) Imagination in practice. *Journal of Medical Ethics* 23, 45–50.

Tanner, C.A., Benner, P., Chesla, C. & Gordon, D. (1996) The phenomenology of knowing the patient. In S. Gordon, P. Benner & N. Noddings (Eds) *Caregiving: Readings in knowledge, practice, ethics & politics* (pp. 203–219). Philadelphia: University of Pennsylvania Press.

Webb, J. & Warwick, C. (1999) Getting it right: The teaching of philosophical health care ethics. *Nurs Ethics* 6(2), 150–156.

White, M.T. (2006) Diagnosing PVS and minimally conscious states: The role of tacit knowledge and intuition. *J Clin Ethics* 17(1), 62–71.

Woods, M. (2005) Nursing ethics education: Are we really delivering the good(s)? *Nurs Ethics* 12(1), 5–18.

Appendix 2
Taking moral action

Megan-Jane Johnstone

Division of Nursing and Midwifery
RMIT University
Melbourne, Australia

Nurses in all areas and at all levels of practice encounter ethical issues in the course of their day-to-day work. When encountering ethical issues in the workplace, nurses have to decide whether to take action and, in the event of deciding to act, what kind of action to take, when, and whether to act alone or in collaboration with others. In addition, as members of a socially relevant profession whose obligations also extend to the broader community, nurses may encounter ethical issues that are not directly related to their day-to-day work or even to the professional domain of nursing as such, but which demand a response by the nursing profession nevertheless (Des Jardin 2001). Issues involving the unjust exploitation and degradation of the natural environment, calling for a ban on nuclear weapons, and fighting for democracy in countries whose political systems are undemocratic, are some examples.

It is well recognised both within and outside the profession of nursing that nursing is a morally responsible and accountable profession. It is further recognised that nurses are individually morally responsible and accountable for their own actions. Related to this, it is generally expected that nurses will take appropriate (moral) action, in the context of their work, to promote the moral interests of those in their care as well as the broader communities in which they live and work. This observation raises three key questions: What is moral action? What qualities must nurses have in order to be effective moral actors in nursing and healthcare contexts? What kind of actions should nurses engage in, and when?

Taking moral action

What is moral action? If a nurse merely thinks about and/or acknowledges his or her moral duty in a given situation, does this count as moral action per se, and, by virtue of the fact, a discharge of that nurse's moral responsibilities in the situation at hand? The short answer to this latter question is 'no'.

The term 'action' may be defined as the state or process of doing something. Moral action, by this view, may be defined as something (i.e. some physical process, preceded by an act of moral will; an occurrence effected by the volition of a human agent) that someone does in order to achieve a desirable moral outcome.

Moral action is not merely a thought about doing something. Rather, moral action is the 'deed done' as it were. It is the physical process that occurs as a direct consequence of a given thought-to-action. For instance, thinking that such-and-such is the right thing to do is not the same as actually doing it. Merely thinking 'I should develop a policy on conscientious objection to be implemented in my workplace' is not the same as actually drafting a policy on conscientious objection, submitting it to the relevant authorities for approval and overseeing its implementation in the workplace once approved. Although obviously closely connected, it is the deed done that ultimately distinguishes a moral action from the mere thought of moral action.

Moral initiative and taking action

'Taking action' in nursing and healthcare contexts – as well as in broader social and political contexts – is not a simple matter. Additionally, contrary to popular views expressed in the nursing literature, neither is it simply a matter of identifying and applying certain moral rules, principles and theories of conduct and taking physical action accordingly. There are other processes that must be taken into consideration.

In the first instance 'taking action' requires moral initiative on the part of the nurse. Moral initiative, in this instance, may be defined as the ability and attitude required to begin or initiate (i.e. without prompting) a moral action designed to achieve a desirable moral end (e.g. the prevention of harm, the promotion of justice). To have the ability and attitude necessary to take moral action without prompting, nurses must have:

> 'an exquisite moral sensibility, "moral knowing" [knowing that and knowing how], moral imagination, life experience, virtue (e.g. compassion, empathy, integrity, care, "decency"), being generally informed (e.g. about law, social and cultural processes, human nature, politics), and a deep personal moral commitment to "doing what is right" ' (Johnstone 1999, p. 429).

In some situations moral initiative may also require nurses to have political savvy as well as enormous moral courage. And, although it should be otherwise, taking moral action may also require moral heroism on the part of the nurse (Johnstone 2002, 2004a, 2004b).

Finally, in order to be able to use their moral initiative and take moral action, nurses must be able to:

- identify correctly the most pertinent ethical issues facing nurses (locally and globally) at a given time
- recognise both the short- and long-term implications of the issues identified for the nursing profession and the individuals, groups and communities it serves
- develop strategies for responding appropriately and effectively to the issues once identified

Related to the above, for moral initiative to succeed it must have as its over-all aim:

- promotion of human well-being and welfare
- balancing the needs and significant moral interests of different people
- making reliable judgments on what constitutes right and wrong conduct and providing sound justification for the decisions and actions taken on the basis of these judgments (Johnstone 2004a)

Individual moral action

Nurses should never underestimate their capacity, as individuals, to achieve good moral outcomes in the contexts in which they live and work. Sometimes what is required of nurses is not some great startling heroic deed, but a 'simple' act of kindness or compassion or integrity or attentiveness toward those in their care or a co-worker. In some contexts it may require little more than a willingness to challenge the status quo – to question and call into question things as they are – to question seriously why something is being done the way it is rather than some other (more effective) way, and then initiating the more effective way.

A nurse's considered moral action can make a significant difference to the life and well-being of another. A notable example of this can be found in the little known case reported in *Telling the Truth about Jerusalem*, written by the internationally reputed sociologist Ann Oakley. In this work, Oakley describes how she was greatly affected by the actions of one nurse. Oakley had been admitted to hospital for treatment of a tumour on her tongue. She writes:

> 'I remember silently crying in front of the consultant the day the tumour was diagnosed. All he said was, "What are you crying about? The treatment won't affect your appearance". My appearance was not what I worried about' (Oakley 1986, p. 182).

Later, a young nurse, entering Oakley's room to collect her lunch tray, noticed she was crying. Instead of removing the tray, the nurse sat down immediately and talked with Oakley for over an hour – something she wasn't supposed to do because Oakley was 'radioactive' on account of a radium implant in her tongue. Oakley discussed her fears and anxieties about the tumour and its treatment. The nurse then went and checked the medical notes and returned to reassure Oakley that she 'would probably be all right' – again doing something she was not supposed to do (i.e. report back Oakley's medical notes) (Oakley 1986, p. 182). Of this experience, Oakley later wrote, 'I never saw this nurse again after I left hospital, but I would like her to know that she was important to my survival' (Oakley 1986, p. 182). Although this incident occurred some years ago, its lessons are still pertinent today.

A more recent (and controversial) example concerns an experienced intensive care nurse assigned to care for a man who was estranged from his identical twin brother and whom he had not seen for several years (Johnstone 2004b). The man's condition was serious and it was evident to all that he was dying. Despite being aware of his deteriorating condition, the man was adamant that 'he did not want any contact with his twin brother' and that 'his twin brother was not to be contacted and told about his condition' (Johnstone 2004b, p. 4). Acting on intuition, the nurse decided, however, to 'respectfully disagree' with her patient's request and to take action to redress the situation at hand. Recognising that time was running out (the man was not expected to live very long), she immediately set in motion a chain of events that resulted in the estranged brothers being happily reunited and reconciled before the ill brother died. Prior to the ill twin's death, both brothers were insistent that the nurse had 'done the right thing' and expressed their deep appreciation for her insights, sensitivity and actions (Johnstone 2004b, p. 4).

There are a range of ordinary, everyday actions that nurses can engage in to promote the moral interests of their patients, such as ensuring patients are treated with fairness and respect, receive relevant information concerning their care and treatment, have their cultural values and beliefs respected, receive adequate pain relief, receive adequate support when 'the system' seems to be failing them, have their (and their loved ones') concerns addressed in a prompt and appropriate manner, and so forth.

Sometimes nurses may have to engage in extraordinary action to achieve good moral outcomes, such as: report unsafe work practices or an impaired co-worker to a supervisor or statutory authority; refuse conscientiously to participate in a certain medical procedure; join an organised strike action or political march. Such action is not without risks to the nurse, however (Johnstone 1994, 2002, 2004a, 2004c). There have been a number of notable cases across the globe where nurses have faced disciplinary proceedings and even court action as a direct consequence of 'taking moral action' (see, for example, Andersen 1990; Fry & Veatch 2006; Hart & Snell 1992; Johnstone 2004a, 2004c; Liddell 1994; Turner 1990, 1992). One such example is the New Zealand Neil Pugmire case.

Neil Pugmire, a registered psychiatric nurse, wrote in confidence to the then Minister of Health outlining concerns he had about New Zealand's mental health legislation and its failure to provide for the compulsory detainment of patients whom responsible health professionals strongly believed were 'very dangerous'. To support his concerns, Pugmire used as an example a named patient whom mental health professionals thought 'was highly likely to commit very serious sexual acts with little boys' if released (Liddell 1994, p. 15). The Minister, however, reputedly took the position that 'mental health legislation should not be used to justify the detention of difficult or dangerous individuals' (Liddell 1994, p. 14). Dissatisfied with this response, Pugmire sent a confidential copy of his letter to a member of the opposition party. This politician subsequently released the letter publicly, but with the patient's name deleted. However, the patient's name was eventually revealed by other sources, thus breaching his confidentiality. Consequently, Pugmire was suspended by his employer for 'serious misconduct' involving the unauthorised disclosure of confidential patient information (Liddell 1994, p. 16).

In some countries, such as those torn apart by political unrest or war, nurses have faced – and continue to face – imprisonment, torture and even death for taking a moral stand and engaging in moral action, such as working to promote human rights (Amnesty International 2000; Johnstone 1988; Welsh 2000). The moral responsibilities of nurses in these countries is disproportionately more burdensome than those carried by other nurses in more peaceful and less threatening political environments. The nursing profession generally has a responsibility to support their colleagues who are living and working in threatening political environments and in which upholding the ethical standards of the profession could result in their untimely deaths. Moral action in this instance might mean nurses globally taking action to promote and protect the moral interests of their colleagues living and working in repressive political environments.

Collective moral action

Nurses can also achieve a great deal by engaging in collective action. Collective action is usually more powerful than individual action and is usually more successful for this reason. It also helps to reduce the vulnerability of individual nurses who, when acting alone, might otherwise be 'martyred' by the system and be left to carry a disproportionate burden of responsibility for taking the moral action they did. It is much more difficult for an organisation to ignore the voices of 100 nurses than it would be for them to ignore the voice of just one nurse. The challenge for the nursing profession, however, is to find and cultivate its collective voice on issues of moral importance.

Nurses leading moral change and development

The nursing profession has not been very successful in getting its collective voice heard or in getting the public, as well as governments, to understand what nursing is about (Buresch & Gordon 2000; Gordon 2005; Johnstone 1999). It is appropriate and timely that nurses locally, nationally and internationally situate themselves to be leaders in – and agents of – moral change and development in health and healthcare domains, and to develop and implement a well-organised political action strategy toward these worthy ends (Des Jardin 2001; Gordon 2005; Johnstone 2004a). As Johnstone has stated, 'There is nothing unprofessional or dishonourable about engaging in lobbying activities, and there is no reason why nurses should not "pick up the gauntlet" [of moral activism]' (Johnstone 1999, p. 439). Moreover, collective action can be very satisfying. As one Australian action lobby collective has pointed out:

> 'Action can be fun. Even when you know that it's mainly symbolic it's still more gratifying to act collectively than to fume privately. Action means getting together with other people to talk things over, finding out that other people have the same concerns that you have, and then taking those concerns to the people in power and publicly demanding that they do something about it' (National Women's Consultative Council 1988, p. 41).

Policy development and reform

An area of particular concern for the nursing profession is that of policy development and reform – including law reform. Nurses worldwide have suffered terrible hardships on account of inappropriate and restrictive government and institutional policies as well as legislation governing the profession and practice of nursing (Des Jardin 2001; Johnstone 1994). Today, despite considerable progress being made in regard to the professionalisation of nursing, nurses continue to carry an enormous burden of responsibility in their areas of practice without the legitimated authority necessary to match it (Johnstone 1994, 2004a). In other words, nurses are responsible for many things but often lack the legal backing necessary to enable them to take the responsible actions expected of them.

The nursing profession has a significant moral interest in researching the inadequacies and deficiencies of institutional and government policies, as well as existing legislation, and actively leading and lobbying for change of those policies and laws that have a negative impact on the ability of nurses to deliver safe, therapeutically effective and ethical nursing care (see, for example, Johnstone & Kanitsaki 2006), and on the overall safety, quality, accessibility and sustainability of available healthcare services.

The nursing profession would also benefit from identifying specific issues for which policy guidelines are needed – such as Do Not Resuscitate (DNR) directives, informed consent, abortion, euthanasia/assisted suicide, conscientious objection, and other related issues. Until policy and law reforms are achieved in these and similar areas, nurses will never be free to practise nursing as they have been taught to practise it, as nursing research suggests it should be practised, and as the public is entitled to have it practised; nor will they be 'free to be moral' – that is, 'free to practise as morally accountable and responsible professionals' (Johnstone 1999).

Where to from here? What should nurses do? The answer to this question is: doing. Doing whatever needs to be done to make healthcare contexts not just morally tolerable but morally excellent. Doing whatever needs to be done to protect people's significant moral interests – their genuine welfare and well-being – and to prevent them from suffering unnecessary harm. Doing whatever needs to be done to achieve satisfactory solutions to the moral disagreements and controversies which may arise among patients, patients' families, friends, lay carers, co-workers, managers and officials in healthcare domains. And doing what needs to be done to promote and protect health and human rights in nursing and related domains.

Nurses cannot be morally passive bystanders to the suffering of others. They are obliged to take a stand and to take moral action when it is within their capacity to do so. For nurses to do otherwise is not only to fail the profession of nursing and the people the profession serves, but to fail themselves.

References

Amnesty International (2000) *Harming the healers: The violation of human rights of health professionals (ACT 75/02/00)*. London: Amnesty International.

Andersen, S. (1990) Patient advocacy and whistle-blowing in nursing: Help for the helpers. *Nursing Forum* 25(3), 5–13.

Buresch, B. & Gordon, S. (2000) *From silence to voice: When nurses know and must communicate to the public*. Ottawa: Canadian Nurses Association.

Des Jardin, K. (2001) Political involvement in nursing – politics, ethics, and strategic action. *AORN* 74(5), 614–615, 617–618, 621–626, 628.

Fry, S.T. & Veatch, R.M. (2006) *Case studies in nursing ethics*, 3rd ed. Boston: Jones & Bartlett, Publishers.

Gordon, S. (2005) *Nursing against the odds: How health care costs cutting, media stereotypes, and medical hubris undermine nurses and patient care*. Ithaca and London: ILR Press, an imprint of Cornell University Press.

Hart, R. & Snell, J. (1992) Dr Cox: The nurse's story. *Nursing Times* 88(41), 19.

Johnstone, M. (1988) Support for Amnesty International: A nursing perspective. *Australian Nurses Journal* 18(3), 10–11.

Johnstone, M. (1994) *Nursing and the injustices of the law*. Sydney: WB Saunders/ Baillière Tindall.

Johnstone, M. (1999) *Bioethics: A nursing perspective*, 3rd ed. Sydney: Harcourt Australia.

Johnstone, M. (2002) Poor working conditions and the capacity of nurses to provide moral care. *Contemporary Nurse* 12(1), 7–15.

Johnstone, M. (2004a) *Bioethics: A nursing perspective*, 4th ed. Sydney: Churchill Livingstone/Elsevier Science.

Johnstone, M. (2004b) *Effective writing for health professionals: A practical guide to getting published*. London/New York: Routledge.

Johnstone, M. (2004c) Patient safety, ethics and whistle blowing: A nursing response to the events at the Campbelltown and Camden Hospitals. *Australian Health Review* 28(1), 13–19.

Johnstone, M. & Kanitsaki, O. (2006) The ethics and practical importance of defining, distinguishing and disclosing nursing errors: a discussion paper. *International Journal of Nursing Studies* 43(3), 367–376.

Liddell, G. (1994) Pugmire and the dilemma of disclosure. *Otago Bioethics Report* 3(2), 14–16.

National Women's Consultative Council (1988) *Women into action*. Canberra: CPN Publications.

Oakley, A. (1986) *Telling the truth about Jerusalem*. Oxford, UK: Basil Blackwell.

Turner, T. (1990) Crushed by the system? *Nursing Times* 86(49), 19.

Turner, T. (1992) The indomitable Mr Pink. *Nursing Times* 88(24), 26–29.

Welsh, J. (2000) Health workers at risk. *The Lancet* 356(9228), 503.

Appendix 3
Glossary

accountability Being answerable to someone for something one has done or for the responsibilities associated with a particular role assumed by the individual. It includes providing an explanation or rationale according to public standards/norms. The standards/norms of legal accountability are specified by licensure requirements and nurse practice acts/legislation; the standards/ norms of moral accountability are specified by codes of ethics and practice standards.

advocacy Active support of an important cause; speaking on behalf of someone else.

allocation of resources The decision-making process by which goods and services are distributed to people. Macro allocation decisions occur at the level of policy and establish how many costs should be used in distribution, which goods and services will be distributed and the process of distribution. Micro allocation decisions occur at the individual level and concern who will receive the goods or services to be distributed.

answerability Giving an account, explaining, or justifying one's actions and/or judgments carried out in a particular role.

applied ethics The use of ethical theory and the methods of ethical analysis to examine ethical questions in the professions, technology use and public policy.

argument A process of reasoning to convince someone of the truth or worth of something. Types of argument include appeals to authority, appeals to consensus, appeals to intuition and dialectical reasoning.

assisted suicide Ending one's own life with the help of another person.

autonomy Ethical principle that obliges one to allow individuals to self-determine their own plans and actions. It entails respecting the personal liberty of individuals and the choices they make, based on their own personal values and beliefs.

beneficence   Ethical principle that obliges one to provide good (promote some-one's welfare, for example).

bioethics   Applied ethics inquiry in the biomedical sciences that attempts to pro-vide moral responses to difficult questions arising in healthcare, technology use and related public policy.

caring   A form of involvement with others that expresses concern about how they are experiencing their world. Often expressed by behaviour that protects and preserves the health, welfare and human dignity of another. A moral duty or obligation for individuals in certain relationships to another (mother/child; nurse/patient; etc.).

code of ethics   A formal statement by a group that establishes and prescribes moral standards and behaviours for members of the group.

collective good   The good or human welfare of groups or populations.

confidentiality   The ethical obligation to keep someone's personal and private information secret or private.

cooperation   A concept of active participation, collaboration and reciprocity with others to obtain or achieve something.

cultural values   Standards of behaviour that derive from a particular cultural group.

emotivism   Ethical theory maintaining that ethical judgments are expressions of one's feelings and desires.

ethical behaviour   Moral behaviour, actions and decisions in response to moral standards, norms.

ethical concept   Mental image, idea or form of abstract thought about ethical responsibility, such as advocacy, accountability, cooperation and caring.

ethical decision making framework   A model of the process of making an ethical decision, highlighting the relevant ethical questions and the moral reasoning involved. A framework represents the approach or process that one might use in making an ethical decision.

ethical issue   Any situation that requires ethical deliberation or ethical deci-sion making, or a conflict of moral values. Examples of ethical issues include abortion, euthanasia, surrogate motherhood, rationing healthcare to the elderly, etc.

ethical practice Nurses' moral behaviour, actions, decisions and ethical decision making in everyday practice.

ethical principle A guide to moral decision making and moral action. Examples include autonomy, beneficence and justice.

ethical sensitivity The ability to recognise values and value conflicts.

ethical theory An integrated body of principles and rules governing choices when values are in conflict. Consequential theories claim that certain acts are right and others are wrong because of their consequences (example, utilitarianism). Nonconsequential theories claim that certain acts are right and others are wrong because of the features of the acts (right-making or wrong-making characteristics) or their conformity (nonconformity) to duty or obligations (example, formalism).

ethics The moral practices, beliefs and standards of individuals and/or groups. Also, a particular form of inquiry about morality, i.e. normative ethics and nonnormative ethics.

etiquette Prescribed requirements for polite social behaviour, actions, decisions and ethical decision making in response to conflicts of moral value.

euthanasia The act of actively or passively killing a person painlessly for reasons of mercy. Active euthanasia is the direct killing or ending of someone's life by any method such as lethal injection or a lethal dose of medication. Passive euthanasia is the withholding or withdrawing of a life-sustaining measure in order to allow a person to die.

fidelity Ethical principle that obliges one to remain faithful to one's commitments, especially the keeping of promises and the protection of confidentiality.

hedonism Theory of ethics maintaining that pleasure or happiness is the highest good.

human dignity Excellence of the human condition. Deeply valued inner sense of well-being and personal worth.

incompetent behaviour Individual behaviour that fails to meet specified standards of the group. Can be caused by physical or mental impairment of the individual's capacities or by ignorance of the standards of the group.

individual good The good or human welfare of the individual person.

intuitionism Ethical theory maintaining that our basic ethical principles and value judgments are intuitive or self-evident. Ethical judgments are true or false, but are not factual and cannot be justified by empirical observation, argument, or reasoning. They are only known through intuition.

justice   Ethical principle that obliges one to treat those who are equal, in relevant respects, in the same manner. When individuals are unequal, in relevant respects, one is obliged to treat them in a fair manner. This means that those who have greater need may justly receive more of a particular resource than those with less need.

moral agency   The capacity for a person to act morally or ethically on his own (moral) authority.

moral character   The perseverance, strength of conviction and courage that enable a person to carry out a plan of moral action that he or she deems imperative.

moral development   A series of stages in which one develops moral reasoning abilities and skills.

moral dilemma   A situation where there are two equally justifiable courses of action or judgments and the individual is uncertain which one to pursue or choose.

moral distress   A situation where the individual knows the right course of action to follow and can morally justify that action but is unable to carry out the action because of one or more constraints. These constraints may include legal rules, institutional policies, lack of decision-making authority and/or lack of recognition of the person's moral agency.

moral ideal   A conception of moral perfection or excellence. A possible state of affairs that is morally desirable.

morality   A set of culturally defined goals and the rules governing how we attain those goals. The goals to be attained include certain dispositions, character traits and/or virtues.

moral motivation   A genuine desire and interest to achieve good moral outcomes. It involves one's sense of moral responsibility and integrity and a commitment to achieving moral ends.

moral reasoning   The cognitive process by which one chooses among one's values in order to come to some decision about one's moral behaviour. This process takes place after recognition of values and value conflicts (ethical sensitivity or moral sensitivity) and usually results in judgment formation or an action (moral behaviour). Synonym: moral judgment.

moral sensitivity   The awareness of situational aspects that affect the welfare and well-being of an individual. It requires insight, intuition, moral knowing, and the ability to recognise the salient moral cues in a situation that indicates that a moral issue is present. Synonym: ethical sensitivity

moral uncertainty   A situation in which the individual recognises that values are in conflict but is uncertain which values they are, or feels uncomfortable about the situation, or does not have full information about the situation.

moral values   Those values ascribed to human actions, behaviours, institutions or character traits.

naturalism   Ethical theory maintaining that ethical judgments are based on natural inclinations and desires given by nature or by God.

nonmaleficence   The ethical obligation to avoid doing harm.

nonmoral values   Those values related to personal preferences, beliefs or matters of taste.

nonnormative ethics   Type of ethics inquiry that investigates the phenomena of moral beliefs and behaviour (descriptive ethics) or analyses the moral language and concepts used in ethics inquiry and the logic of moral justification (metaethics).

normative ethics   Type of ethics inquiry that examines standards (norms) or criteria for right or wrong conduct. Using ethical theories such as utilitarianism, naturalism, formalism and pragmatism, it defends a system of moral principles and rules to determine which actions are right or wrong.

nursing ethics   The philosophical analysis of (1) the moral phenomena found in nursing practice, (2) the moral language and ethical foundations of nursing practice, and (3) the ethical judgments made by nurses. Also, proposals about the normative aims or content of nursing practice.

paternalism   The overriding of individual choice or actions in order to provide benefit to that individual or to prevent harm from occurring to the individual. Paternalistic actions may be morally justified when the benefits realised are great and the harms avoided are significant.

personal values   Moral and nonmoral beliefs, attitudes or standards considered important to the individual and that form a basis for his or her behaviour and choices.

privacy   State of being private; nondisclosure of the self.

professional values   Moral and nonmoral beliefs, attitudes or standards that are derived from one's professional group.

rationing   Restricting certain provisions (such as food, treatments or medications) or resources (such as healthcare services, nursing care, organs or technologies) by some method of distribution.

responsibility   Obligation to carry out duties associated with a particular role assumed by the individual.

rights   A just claim that a person has and that ought to be protected. Legal rights are valid claims recognised by the legal system. Moral rights are valid claims derived from customs, traditions or ideals which may be upheld or protected by the law.

right to health   A morally just claim or entitlement to freedom from illness, debilitating disease or risk of illness or disease. A negative right to health is a moral right not to have one's health endangered by the actions of others. A positive right to health is a moral right to obtain resources or services to guarantee a state free of illness or debilitating disease. A right to healthcare is a positive moral right to goods and services that will maintain and improve whatever state of health one already has.

stoicism   A theory of ethics maintaining indifference to pleasure, the repression of emotion and submission of the will without complaint.

torture   The systematic and deliberate infliction of acute pain in any form by one person on another in order to accomplish a purpose against the will of the tortured person.

unethical behaviour   Individual behaviour that knowingly and willingly violates fundamental norms of ethical conduct toward others.

value(s)   A standard or quality that is esteemed, desired, considered important or has worth or merit. Values are expressed by behaviours or standards that a person endorses or tries to maintain. Values are organised into a hierarchical system of importance to the individual.

value conflict   Opposition or clash among values considered important by an individual or a group.

veracity   Ethical principle that obliges one to tell the truth and not to lie or deceive others.

virtue   A disposition (such as honesty or kindness) or trait (such as conscientiousness) that is valued and is acquired, in part, by teaching and practice and perhaps by grace. A disposition or habit to undertake certain types of actions in certain types of situations in accordance with moral obligation or moral ideals is often called moral virtue.

Appendix 4
ICN Code of Ethics

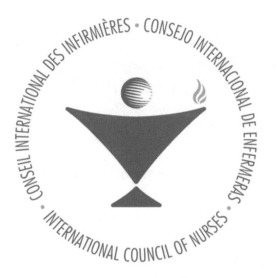

The ICN CODE OF ETHICS
FOR NURSES

Copyright © 2006 by ICN – International Council for Nurses, 3, place Jean-Marteau, CH-1201 Geneva (Switzerland)

ISBN: 92-95040-41-4

The ICN Code of Ethics for Nurses

An international code of ethics for nurses was first adopted by the International Council of Nurses (ICN) in 1953. It has been revised and reaffirmed at various times since, most recently with this review and revision completed in 2005.

Preamble

Nurses have four fundamental responsibilities: to promote health, to prevent illness, to restore health and to alleviate suffering. The need for nursing is universal.

Inherent in nursing is respect for human rights, including cultural rights, the right to life and choice, to dignity and to be treated with respect. Nursing care is respectful of and unrestricted by considerations of age, colour, creed, culture, disability or illness, gender, sexual orientation, nationality, politics, race or social status.

Nurses render health services to the individual, the family and the community and co-ordinate their services with those of related groups.

THE CODE

The *ICN Code of Ethics for Nurses* has four principal elements that outline the standards of ethical conduct.

Elements of the Code

1. Nurses and people

The nurse's primary professional responsibility is to people requiring nursing care.

In providing care, the nurse promotes an environment in which the human rights, values, customs and spiritual beliefs of the individual, family and community are respected.

The nurse ensures that the individual receives sufficient information on which to base consent for care and related treatment.

The nurse holds in confidence personal information and uses judgement in sharing this information.

The nurse shares with society the responsibility for initiating and supporting action to meet the health and social needs of the public, in particular those of vulnerable populations.

The nurse also shares responsibility to sustain and protect the natural environment from depletion, pollution, degradation and destruction.

2. Nurses and practice

The nurse carries personal responsibility and accountability for nursing practice, and for maintaining competence by continual learning.

The nurse maintains a standard of personal health such that the ability to provide care is not compromised.

The nurse uses judgement regarding individual competence when accepting and delegating responsibility.

The nurse at all times maintains standards of personal conduct which reflect well on the profession and enhance public confidence.

The nurse, in providing care, ensures that use of technology and scientific advances are compatible with the safety, dignity and rights of people.

3. Nurses and the profession

The nurse assumes the major role in determining and implementing acceptable standards of clinical nursing practice, management, research and education.

The nurse is active in developing a core of research-based professional knowledge.

The nurse, acting through the professional organisation, participates in creating and maintaining safe, equitable social and economic working conditions in nursing.

4. Nurses and co-workers

The nurse sustains a co-operative relationship with co-workers in nursing and other fields.

The nurse takes appropriate action to safeguard individuals, families and communities when their care is endangered by a co-worker or any other person.

Suggestions for use of the *ICN Code of Ethics for Nurses*

The *ICN Code of Ethics for Nurses* is a guide for action based on social values and needs. It will have meaning only as a living document if applied to the realities of nursing and health care in a changing society.

To achieve its purpose the *Code* must be understood, internalised and used by nurses in all aspects of their work. It must be available to students and nurses throughout their study and work lives.

Applying the elements of the *ICN Code of Ethics for Nurses*

The four elements of the *ICN Code of Ethics for Nurses*: nurses and people, nurses and practice, nurses and the profession, and nurses and co-workers, give a framework for the standards of conduct. The following chart will assist nurses to translate the standards into action. Nurses and nursing students can therefore:

- Study the standards under each element of the *Code*.
- Reflect on what each standard means to you. Think about how you can apply ethics in your nursing domain: practice, education, research or management.
- Discuss the *Code* with co-workers and others.
- Use a specific example from experience to identify ethical dilemmas and standards of conduct as outlined in the *Code*. Identify how you would resolve the dilemma.
- Work in groups to clarify ethical decision making and reach a consensus on standards of ethical conduct.
- Collaborate with your national nurses' association, co-workers, and others in the continuous application of ethical standards in nursing practice, education, management and research.

Element of the Code #1: NURSES AND PEOPLE		
Practitioners and managers	**Educators and researchers**	**National nurses' associations**
Provide care that respects human rights and is sensitive to the values, customs and beliefs of all people.	In curriculum include references to human rights, equity, justice, solidarity as the basis for access to care.	Develop position statements and guidelines that support human rights and ethical standards.
Provide continuing education in ethical issues.	Provide teaching and learning opportunities for ethical issues and decision making.	Lobby for involvement of nurses in ethics review committees.
Provide sufficient information to permit informed consent and the right to choose or refuse treatment.	Provide teaching/learning opportunities related to informed consent.	Provide guidelines, position statements and continuing education related to informed consent.
Use recording and information management systems that ensure confidentiality.	Introduce into curriculum concepts of privacy and confidentiality.	Incorporate issues of confidentiality and privacy into a national code of ethics for nurses.
Develop and monitor environmental safety in the workplace.	Sensitise students to the importance of social action in current concerns.	Advocate for safe and health environment.

Element of the Code #2: NURSES AND PRACTICE		
Practitioners and managers	**Educators and researchers**	**National nurses' associations**
Establish standards of care and a work setting that promotes safety and quality care.	Provide teaching/learning opportunities that foster life long learning and competence for practice.	Provide access to continuing education, through journals, conferences, distance education, etc.
Establish systems for professional appraisal, continuing education and systematic renewal of licensure to practice.	Conduct and disseminate research that shows links between continual learning and competence to practice.	Lobby to ensure continuing education opportunities and quality care standards.
Monitor and promote the personal health of nursing staff in relation to their competence for practice.	Promote the importance of personal health and illustrate its relation to other values.	Promote healthy lifestyles for nursing professionals. Lobby for healthy workplaces and services for nurses.

Element of the Code #3: NURSES AND THE PROFESSION		
Practitioners and managers	**Educators and researchers**	**National nurses' associations**
Set standards for nursing practice, research, education and management.	Provide teaching/learning opportunities in setting standards for nursing practice, research, education and management.	Collaborate with others to set standards for nursing education, practice, research and management.
Foster workplace support of the conduct, dissemination and utilisation of research related to nursing and health.	Conduct, disseminate and utilise research to advance the nursing profession.	Develop position statements, guidelines and standards related to nursing research.
Promote participation in national nurses' associations so as to create favourable socio-economic conditions for nurses.	Sensitise learners to the importance of professional nursing associations.	Lobby for fair social and economic working conditions in nursing. Develop position statements and guidelines in workplace issues.

Element of the Code #4: NURSES AND CO-WORKERS		
Practitioners and managers	**Educators and researchers**	**National nurses' associations**
Create awareness of specific and overlapping functions and the potential for interdisciplinary tensions.	Develop understanding of the roles of other workers.	Stimulate co-operation with other related disciplines.
Develop workplace systems that support common professional ethical values and behaviour.	Communicate nursing ethics to other professions.	Develop awareness of ethical issues of other professions.
Develop mechanisms to safeguard the individual, family or community when their care is endangered by health care personnel.	Instil in learners the need to safeguard the individual, family or community when care is endangered by health care personnel.	Provide guidelines, position statements and discussion fora related to safeguarding people when their care is endangered by health care personnel.

Dissemination of the *ICN Code of Ethics for Nurses*

To be effective the *ICN Code of Ethics for Nurses* must be familiar to nurses. We encourage you to help with its dissemination to schools of nursing, practising nurses, the nursing press and other mass media. The *Code* should also be disseminated to other health professions, the general public, consumer and policy-making groups, human rights organisations and employers of nurses.

Glossary of terms used in the *ICN Code of Ethics for Nurses*

Co-worker Other nurses and other health and non-health related workers and professionals.

Co-operative relationship A professional relationship based on collegial and reciprocal actions, and behaviour that aim to achieve certain goals.

Family A social unit composed of members connected through blood, kinship, emotional or legal relationships.

Nurse shares with society A nurse, as a health professional and a citizen, initiates and supports appropriate action to meet the health and social needs of the public.

Personal health Mental, physical, social and spiritual well-being of the nurse.

Personal information Information obtained during professional contact that is private to an individual or family, and which, when disclosed, may violate the right to privacy, cause inconvenience, embarrassment, or harm to the individual or family.

Related groups Other nurses, health care workers or other professionals providing service to an individual, family or community and working toward desired goals.

Index